OXFORD MONOGRAPHS ON MEDICAL GENETICS

The Distribution of the Human Immunoglobulin Allotypes

ARTHUR G. STEINBERG and
CHARLES E. COOK

*Department of Biology, Case Western Reserve University,
Cleveland, Ohio*

Oxford New York Toronto
OXFORD UNIVERSITY PRESS
1981

Oxford University Press, Walton Street, Oxford OX2 6DP

OXFORD LONDON GLASGOW
NEW YORK TORONTO MELBOURNE WELLINGTON
KUALA LUMPUR SINGAPORE JAKARTA HONG KONG TOKYO
DELHI BOMBAY CALCUTTA MADRAS KARACHI
NAIROBI DAR ES SALAAM CAPE TOWN

British Library Cataloguing in Publication Data
Steinberg, Arthur Gerald
The distribution of the human immunoglobulin
allotypes. — (Oxford monographs on medical
genetics).
1. Blood groups – Statistics
2. Immunoglobulins
I. Title II. Cook, Charles E III. Series
612'.11822 QP98 79–41199
ISBN 0–19–261181–X

Phototypeset in V.I.P. Times by
Western Printing Services Ltd, Bristol
Printed in Great Britain
at the University Press, Oxford
by Eric Buckley
Printer to the University

|| ||

4

THE UNIVERSITY OF LIVERPOOL
HAROLD COHEN LIBRARY

CONDITIONS OF BORROWING

Members of Council, members and retired members of the University staff, and students registered with the University for higher degrees — 20 volumes for one month. All other readers entitled to borrow — 6 volumes for 14 days in term or for the vacation.

Books may be recalled after one week for the use of another reader.

OXFORD MEDICAL PUBLICATIONS

The Distribution of the Human Immunoglobulin Allotypes

Preface

I have long considered publishing a monograph on the distribution of the Gm and Inv groups. Indeed, a first draft was written in 1970, but it was not developed into a form suitable for publication. Gm and Inv data continued to accumulate and we continued to summarize them, but other activities always seemed to intrude and to cause a delay in the resumption of work on the monograph. Its completion is due in large measure to Arthur Mourant, who urged me to complete it when I visited him several years ago. He committed me to complete it by stating in the preface to the second edition of his splendid, indeed classic, book *The distribution of the human blood groups* that I was preparing the monograph.

Although population geneticists, anthropologists, and others are aware of the Gm and Inv groups, it has long been clear to me that, through no fault of theirs, they have not utilized these allotypes in their analyses to the extent that the allotypes should

and can be used. The data are published in many different journals and often in journals which are not widely read. In addition, they are frequently 'buried' in the body of an article and not indicated in the title of the paper nor in abstracts. Review articles have helped, but they cover broad areas, are greatly condensed, and, because of space limitations, do not provide enough data to help those who would make use of population data in their work.

It is my hope that this monograph will provide investigators with easy access to the data and that, as a result, many more investigators will utilize them in their work, and that some will undertake to study the human immunoglobulin allotypes in their laboratories.

Cleveland, Ohio   A.G.S.
October 1979

v

Acknowledgements

Many fine students and post-doctoral Fellows have worked on earlier unpublished compilations of the data. They are too numerous to mention individually. Their names will be found as co-authors among the references. We must, however, mention three individuals who were most active in the early stages of this project, namely, Drs Trefor Jenkins, Thaddeus Kurczynski, and Angus Muir. Their help as well as that of all the others is gratefully acknowledged.

The work in this laboratory was supported in part by grant number GM 07214 from the National Institute of General Medical Sciences of the US Public Health Service.

Contents

Inv tables

Gm maps

Inv maps

INDEXES

1 Introduction

Morphological characters have long been used to classify human beings into races. Mayr (1963), in his excellent book *Animal species and evolution*, states that as early as 1758 Linnaeus classified humans into four living races on the basis of morphological characters. Almost 160 years elapsed before a non-morphological character, the ABO blood types, was applied to human classification (Hirschfeld and Hirschfeld 1919). (The name is usually spelled Hirszfeld, but it is spelled as shown in the 1919 paper.) Twenty years later, Boyd (1939) could publish all the known population data for the blood groups in a brief monograph, and more importantly the data were confined to only two blood-group systems, ABO and MN. Mourant's classic first edition of *The distribution of the human blood groups* (1954) followed Boyd's summary by only 15 years, but by this time eight other blood-group systems and several non-blood-group characters had been sufficiently tested to warrant analysis. The progress since then has been astounding and, to use a trite phrase, 'explosive'. Thus Eloise Giblett discussed in her remarkable book *Genetic markers in human blood* (1969) eleven variants other than blood types that had been and are being used today in human population studies. Only seven years later, in the second edition of Mourant's book, now called *The distribution of the human blood groups and other polymorphisms* (Mourant, Kopeć, and Domaniewska-Sobczak 1976), he presented population data for 16 blood-group systems, 14 plasma-protein systems, 16 red cell enzyme systems, and three other polymorphisms. Two major systems were omitted, by choice, i.e. the immunoglobulin polymorphisms (Gm, Am, Inv (also called Km)) and the HLA cellular antigens.

Many of the systems reviewed by Mourant *et al.* (1976) have been used to characterize human populations, but none of them can do so individually. This distinction is presently limited to the Gm groups, but recent work indicates that the HLA groups may prove to be equally effective (reviewed by McMichael and McDevitt (1977) and by several other authors in *Br. med. Bull.* **34**(3) (1978)). They suffer in comparison with the Gm groups, however, in that the test is more cumbersome and in that very many more reagents are required.

The difference among the human races for all polymorphic systems other than the Gm system are *quantitative*; i.e., with rare exceptions, the antigens are polymorphic in all races. As will be shown later, the difference among races in the Gm system are *qualitative*; i.e. some haplotypes are absent from or confined to certain races. This may prove to be true for some haplotypes in the HLA system also, but the necessary data are not yet available.

Despite their obvious usefulness for population studies (Steinberg 1969) and their demonstrated usefulness for many immunological problems, the immunoglobulin allotypes are studied by remarkably few people. A major reason is that the reagents are not readily available. It is surprising that commercial distributors of antisera have not undertaken to supply these reagents.

The Gm allotypes

Grubb (1956) discovered the first Gm antigen in the course of determining, by means of the Coombs inhibition test, the immunoglobulin G (IgG) levels in the serum of patients with acquired hypogammaglobulinemia. The serum of one patient caused red blood cells (RBC) coated with an incomplete anti-serum, anti-D in the Rh system, to agglutinate. Grubb demonstrated that such agglutinating ability was relatively common in serum from patients with rheumatoid arthritis, and that sera from some donors could inhibit the agglutination when they were mixed with the agglutinating serum. He and Laurell (1956) showed that the ability to inhibit the agglutination is genetically determined and that the inhibitor is located in the gamma globulin fraction of serum. They called the inhibiting sera Gm(a+) and the non-inhibiting sera Gm(a−). Gm stands for gammaglobulin. The Gm antigens are allotypes, i.e. soluble antigens not present in all members of a species (Oudin 1966).

As the reader will have gathered from the foregoing, the Gm test is an agglutination inhibition test. The antigen (Ag)-antibody (Ab) complex is soluble, hence an indicator for the reaction is needed; e.g. red blood cells (RBC) coated with an incomplete Ab. The incomplete Ab is usually anti-D of the Rh system, but any incomplete Ab may be used. The incomplete Ab is IgG and, to be useful, must carry the Gm antigen against which the anti-Gm antiserum is active.

The test system may be outlined as follows:

	Agglutination
RBC[1] suspended in normal saline + anti-D[2] → SRBC[3]	−
Control 1. Anti-allotype + saline + SRBC	+
Control 2. Anti-allotype + known positive serum + SRBC	−
Control 3. Anti-allotype + known negative serum + SRBC	+
Control 4. Serum to be tested + saline + SRBC	− or +
Test Anti-allotype + serum to be tested + SRBC	+ or −

[1]Red blood cells; [2]IgG antibody against the D antigen of the Rh system; [3]Sensitized RBC.

The controls function as follows:

Control 1 is designed to show that the RBC are adequately coated and that the anti-allotype antiserum is active.
Controls 2 and 3 are used to establish that the test is working.
Control 4 indicates whether the serum to be tested has an anti-IgG antibody. If agglutination occurs the serum has an anti-IgG Ab and it must be removed (by dialysing against cold distilled water or by heating at 63 °C for 10 minutes) before the test can be performed.

Controls 1, 2, and 3 need be run only once for a set of tests for a given allotype. Control 4 must be run for each sample to be tested.

The test (last line) is negative if the cells agglutinate in the presence of the serum (i.e. the serum lacks the allotype detected by the anti-allotype antiserum); the test is positive if the cells do not agglutinate in the presence of the serum (i.e. the serum has the allotype detected by the anti-allotype antiserum).

Anti-D antisera are almost invariably $\gamma 1$ or $\gamma 3$ or both, hence they are not useful for determining Gm(23) which is on the $\gamma 2$ chain. Tests for Gm(23) are done by attaching a G2 myeloma protein that is Gm(23) to RBC by means of chromic chloride (Gold and Fudenberg 1967) or some other method.

The demonstration by Ropartz, Lenoir, Hemet, and Rivat (1960) that anti-Gm antibodies may be found in normal sera and that these antibodies are monospecific provided a means for finding antibodies against many more antigens in the Gm system (reviewed in Grubb 1970). Their work led also to the discovery of the Inv system (Ropartz, Lenoir, and Rivat 1961; Steinberg, Wilson, and Lanset 1962).

The Gm antigens are located on the heavy (H) chains of the IgG subclasses. Their subclass distribution, nomenclature, and year of discovery are presented in Table 1. The reader is referred to Grubb's monograph (1970) for further details about these antigens.

Unfortunately more than one system of nomenclature is in use. The major difference between the systems concerns the use of letters, with or without numbers, or simply numbers to designate the allotypes. We prefer the latter system. A panel that met in Rouen (*Am. J. hum. Genet.* **29**:117–20, 1977) suggested that the nomenclature indicate the IgG heavy chain subclass carrying the allotype. For example, the Gm allotypes 1, 2, 3, and 17 are carried by $\gamma 1$ heavy chains. The panel recommended that these be written G1m(1), G1m(2), etc., rather than Gm(1), Gm(2), etc. Similarly, the panel recommended that the allotypes on the $\gamma 3$ chain be written G3m(5), etc. The panel suggested also that the haplotypes be written as $Gm^{1,17;5,13,14}$ if Gm(23), which is on $\gamma 2$, has not been tested for, or $Gm^{1,17;\cdots;5,13,14}$ if Gm(23) has been tested for but is not present, rather than $Gm^{1,5,13,14,17}$ for both cases, as the WHO 1965 working group suggested. The WHO (1965) numerical system (Table 1) is used in this monograph for simplicity of presentation. The custom of listing allotypes tested for and recording only positive reactions is followed throughout.

Each usual haplotype of the Gm system has at least one allotype representing the $\gamma 1$ chain and at least one representing the $\gamma 3$ chain. Since the $\gamma 2$ chain has only one known allotype (Gm(23)), it is not always represented in a haplotype by a known allotype. No allotypes are known on the $\gamma 4$ chain.

At a time when reagents for only Gm(1), Gm(2), Gm(5), and Gm(6) were available, Steinberg, Giles, and Stauffer (1960*a*); and Steinberg, Stauffer, and Fudenberg (1960*b*) showed that the races may be distinguished by their distinct haplotype arrays. Work with subsequently discovered allotypes has confirmed and extended these findings. It seems safe to predict that more extensive studies with Gm(23) located on $\gamma 2$, and with the A2m allotypes on αA_2 (see below), will make these distinctions sharper.

Reagents are readily available only for allotypes Gm(1), Gm(2), Gm(3), and Gm(5). Reagents for the remaining allotypes are available in only a few centres. Hence, tests of serum samples are usually incomplete. At present, sera are routinely tested in this laboratory for Gm(1,2,3,5,6,10,11,13,14, 17,21,24,26). When such tests are done, the haplotypes commonly present in each of several races are those listed in Table 2. Note that the allotypes are listed in numerical sequence and recall that Gm(1), Gm(2), Gm(3), and Gm(17) are on $\gamma 1$ and that all other allotypes listed in Table 2 are on $\gamma 3$.

The Gm allotypes within a race show complete linkage

Table 1 Nomenclature of the IgG allotypes currently testable

IgG Heavy chain subclass	WHO (1965) Nomenclature updated[1]		Year of discovery
	Numeric	Alphameric	
$\gamma 1$	Gm (1)	Gm (a)	1956
	(2)	(x)	1959
	(3)	(f)	1963
	(17)	(z)	1967
$\gamma 2$	Gm (23)	(n)	1966
$\gamma 3$	Gm (5)	(b1)	1959
	(6)	(c3)	1960
	(10)	(b5)	1963
	(11)	(b0)	1963
	(13)	(b3)	1965
	(14)	(b4)	1965
	(15)	(s)	1966
	(16)	(t)	1966
	(21)	(g)	1966
	(24)	(c5)	1967
	(26)	(u)	1973
	(27)	(v)	1974
	(28)	none	1978

[1]A group that met in Rouen in 1974 suggested that the heavy chain subclass carrying the allotype be indicated in the name of the allotype, i.e. G1m(1) rather than Gm(1).

disequilibrium. Thus, in Caucasoids with no racial admixture the $\gamma 1$ allotypes Gm(1), Gm(2), and Gm(17) occur with the $\gamma 3$ allotype Gm(21) and, with rare exceptions, they do not occur with any of the remaining $\gamma 3$ allotypes (Table 2). All Mongoloids have Gm(1), and it may or may not occur with Gm(21). Relatively few Mongoloids have Gm(2), but in Mongoloids as in Caucasoids Gm(2), when present, occurs with Gm(21) but not with other $\gamma 3$ allotypes. Similarly, in Mongoloids, the $\gamma 1$ allotype Gm(17) does not occur with $\gamma 3$ allotypes Gm(5) and Gm(14), while the $\gamma 1$ allotype Gm(3) always occurs with Gm(5) and Gm(14). Similar linkage disequilibria may be noted among the haplotypes of the other races listed in Table 2.

The Gm allotypes have been used extensively in the analysis of the structure of the γ chain and in the analysis of the relation of antigens to the tertiary and quaternary structure of the molecule. These data will not be reviewed here because they are not pertinent to this monograph. The interested reader will find details in reviews by Giblett (1969), Steinberg (1969), and Natvig and Kunkel (1973).

The Inv(Km) allotypes

The panel that met in Rouen suggested that Inv be changed to Km so that the names of all of the allotype systems will start with a letter indicating the chain carrying the allotypes and end in 'm' for consistency. We have retained Inv for historical reasons, because essentially all the sources of data for this analysis used Inv.

The Inv allotypes (Inv(1), Inv(2), and Inv(3)) are carried by the κ chain of Ig (Terry, Fahey, and Steinberg 1965) and are inherited via three alleles, Inv^1, $Inv^{1,2}$, and Inv^3, hence Inv(2) does not occur in the absence of Inv(1).

The molecular explanation is that Inv(2) requires Ala at residue 153 and Leu at residue 191 (Eu numbering) (Steinberg, Milstein, McLaughlin, and Solomon 1974; Milstein, Steinberg,

Table 2 Gm haplotypes commonly present in each of several races[1]

Race	Haplotypes
Caucasoid	(1,17,21,26), (1,2,17,21,26), (3,5,10,11,13,14,26)
Negroid	(1,5,10,11,13,14,17,26), (1,5,10,11,14,17,26), (1,5,6,11,17,24,26), (1,5,6,10,11,14,17,26)
Mongoloid	(1,17,21,26), (1,2,17,21,26), (1,10,11,13,17)[2], (1,3,5,10,11,13,14,26)
Ainu	(1,17,21,26), (1,2,17,21,26), (1,10,11,13,17)[2], (2,17,21,26)
Khoisan	
San (Bushmen)	(1,17,21,26), (1,10,11,13,17)[2], (1,5,10,11,13,14,17,26), (1,5,13,14,17,21,26)[3], (1,5,11,17,26)
Khoikhoi (Hottentots)	(1,2,17,21,26), (1,5,10,11,14,17,26), (1,10,11,13,17)[2], (1,5,10,11,13,14,17,26)
Pygmy	(1,5,6,11,17,24,26), (1,5,10,11,13,14,17,26)
Micronesian	(1,17,21,26), (1,3,5,10,11,13,14,26)
Melanesian	
New Guinea	(1,17,21,26), (1,2,17,21,26), (1,3,5,10,11,13,14,26), (1,5,10,11,13,14,17,26)
Bougainville	(1,17,21,26), (1,2,17,21,26), (1,3,5,10,11,13,14,26)

[1]When tested for Gm(1,2,3,5,6,10,11,13,14,17,21,24,26).
[2]When tests for Gm(15) and Gm(16) are done the haplotype is $Gm^{1,10,11,13,15,16,17}$ among Mongoloids and Ainu, but it may be also $Gm^{1,10,11,13,15,17}$ among the Khoisan.
[3]Not tested for Gm(10) and Gm(11). Gm(10) is probably present, but Gm(11) may not be.

McLaughlin, and Solomon 1974). Substitution of Val for Ala at residue 153 leads to loss of Inv(2) activity, but not of Inv(1) activity, while substitution of Val for Leu at residue 191 leads to loss of both activities and the acquisition of Inv(3) activity.

The Inv locus is not less than 30 centimorgans from the Gm loci (Steinberg and Matsumoto 1964), and by inference is equally removed from A2m locus (see later). The Inv allotypes are determined by an agglutination inhibition test similar to that described for Gm. The anti-D serum must carry a κ light chain with the appropriate Inv antigen on it.

Antisera to detect Inv(2) and Inv(3) are in very short supply; therefore virtually all population samples have been tested for Inv(1) only. This is unfortunate, because it prevents the determination of the frequency of the rare Inv^1 allele (Ropartz, Rousseau, Rivat, Baitsch, Ritter, Pinkerton, and Mermod 1964) and the finding of samples negative for all three allotypes (Steinberg et al. 1962).

Virtually all populations thus far studied are polymorphic for Inv(1) and therefore presumably for Inv(2) and for Inv(3). Hence the differences among populations are quantitative and not qualitative as they are for Gm.

The A2m allotypes

The A2m allotype on $\alpha2$ was discovered independently by two groups of investigators (Vyas and Fudenberg 1969; Kunkel, Smith, Joslin, Natvig, and Litwin 1969). Another allotype on $\alpha2$, A2m(2) was reported by van Loghem, Wang, and Shuster (1973). It acts as an allele of A2m(1) and, as is usual for allotypes, the alleles are inherited as codominants.

Since there are no incomplete anti-RBC antigen antibodies that are IgA$_2$, tests for these allotypes require that RBC be coated with an IgA2 myeloma protein using chromic chloride (Gold and Fudenberg 1967). The test is similar to the Gm and Inv tests in all other aspects. The anti-A2m allotype antibodies are not readily available and only a few population samples have been tested. These have demonstrated quantitative differences in the frequencies of the allotypes among the races.

The A2m locus is closely linked to the Gm loci (Kunkel et al. 1969; van Loghem et al. 1973) and therefore it is not likely to be linked to the Inv locus (see above). There is linkage disequilibrium between the Gm allotypes and the A2m allotypes (Kunkel et al. 1969; van Loghem et al. 1973; Schanfield, Herzog, and Fudenberg 1975).

3

2 Gm haplotypes commonly present in various races

A summary of the Gm haplotypes commonly present in each of the races for which data are available is presented in Table 2 (p. 3). What follows is a review of the data leading to the compilation of the Table.

Australian aborigines

The data for the Australian Aborigines will be found in Tables I-1 to I-4, inclusive. Aborigines from the Western Desert and from the Central region of the Northern Territory have haplotypes $Gm^{1,17,21}$ and $Gm^{1,2,17,21}$ only. Those from more northern regions have $Gm^{1,5,13,14,17}$ in addition to the other haplotypes. There is good reason to believe that the $Gm^{1,5,13,14,17}$ haplotype was acquired through admixture with Melanesians from southern Papua New Guinea (Steinberg and Kirk 1970). We conclude, therefore, that the basic haplotype array for Australian Aborigines is $Gm^{1,17,21}$ and $Gm^{1,2,17,21}$.

Tests for Gm(23) (Table I-4) indicate that among the Aborigines of the Western Desert fewer than 3 per cent of the $Gm^{1,17,21}$ haplotypes have Gm(23), and that 0 to 17 per cent of the $Gm^{1,2,17,21}$ haplotypes have Gm(23). Over 90 per cent of the $Gm^{1,5,10,11,13,14,17}$ haplotypes have Gm(23). The low frequency of occurrence of Gm(23) with the $Gm^{1,17,21}$ haplotype is comparable to the situation in other races.

The haplotypes common to the Australian Aborigines ($Gm^{1,17,21}$ and $Gm^{1,2,17,21}$) are common among Caucasoids, Mongoloids, Oceanic peoples, and the Khoisan (with $Gm^{1,17,21}$ confined to the San, and $Gm^{1,2,17,21}$ confined to the Khoikhoi). Only Negroids fail to have either of these haplotypes. Thus while the Gm data serve to indicate the already known racial uniqueness of the Aborigines, such data do not help to explain the origin of these peoples.

Ainu

The racial origin of the Ainu is obscure. They resemble Mongoloids in some physical and genetic polymorphic blood characters, but in other characters they are clearly different (Omoto 1972). They resemble Caucasoids sufficiently to have led Simmons, Graydon, Semple, and Kodama (1953) to call them Proto-Caucasoid. The Gm data suggest a much closer relationship to Mongoloids than to Caucasoids, and this is consistent with data from other polymorphisms (Omoto 1972). At any rate, it is clear that the Ainu form a distinct race.

There have been only three studies of the Gm allotypes among the Ainu, and in each case the samples came from the south-western region of Hokkaido (Tables II-1–3). None of the populations sampled was free of Japanese admixture; hence there is some doubt about whether certain haplotypes are of Ainu or Japanese origin. It is certain that the Ainu have $Gm^{2,17,21}$ and $Gm^{1,13,15,16,17}$ but neither population nor family data have provided conclusive evidence concerning the presence of $Gm^{1,2,17,21}$. The three sets of data may be explained with or without this haplotype. If $Gm^{1,2,17,21}$ is present, it probably was acquired by admixture with the Japanese. $Gm^{1,3,5,13,14}$ is present in such low frequency that it most likely was acquired by admixture with Japanese. The Ainu are the only race other than the Caucasoids to have a haplotype lacking Gm(1). The $Gm^{2,17,21}$ haplotype has a frequency of about 15 per cent so that only about 2 per cent of the Ainu lack Gm(1). This is much lower than the frequency of Gm(−1) (∼ 49 per cent) among Caucasoids. The Ainu have not been tested for Gm(23).

Caucasoids

Sera from Caucasoids have been studied for a great variety of Gm allotypes (Tables III-1 to III-24, inclusive). Unfortunately, Gm(23), the sole allotype on the $\gamma 2$ chain, has been studied only in samples from Holland, from Ferrara in Italy, from Sardinia (Table III-17), and from Gypsies of unknown origin (Table III-21). The Sardinian and Gypsy populations have considerable admixture with other races, hence they cannot serve as representative Caucasoid populations.

The haplotypes commonly present among Caucasoids of unmixed ancestry (in order of decreasing frequency) are $Gm^{3,5,10,11,13,14,26}$, $Gm^{1,17,21,26}$, and $Gm^{1,2,17,21,26}$ when tested for Gm(1,2,3,5,6,10,11,13,14,15,16,17,21,24,26). No population tested for precisely this array of antigens is included in this monograph, but data from various studies, including unpublished data in our laboratory, establish the above haplotypes. Tests with Gm (23) show that it is almost invariably associated with the $Gm^{3,5,10,11,13,14,26}$ haplotype to yield a $Gm^{3,5,10,11,13,14,23,26}$ haplotype, in addition to the former. Among the Dutch (Table III-17, p. 57), the relative frequencies of these two haplotypes are approximately 1:2. Two individuals among the Gypsies had the phenotype Gm(1,17,21,23), establishing that Gm(23) occurs in a $Gm^{1,17,21,23}$ haplotype. There is evidence in this population that a $Gm^{1,10,11,13,17,23}$ haplotype may occur, but the $Gm^{1,10,11,13,17}$ haplotype is not characteristic of Caucasoids.

The $Gm^{1,3}$ haplotype, or $Gm^{1,3,21}$ haplotype, when tested for Gm(21), has been found at polymorphic frequencies among the French (Table III-7, p. 39), Italians (Table III-7, p. 391, Parsi and Irani (Table III-13, pp. 45, 46), and Kurdish Jews (Table III-23, p. 64); this haplotype has been found at non-polymorphic frequencies among Germans (Table III-5, pp. 33). The significance of this finding is not apparent, but we point out that the $Gm^{1,3,21}$ haplotype can arise from the relatively common $Gm^{1,17,21}$ haplotype by a substitution of arginine for lysine at residue 214 in the $\gamma 1$ chain of IgG and that this requires a change from A to G in the second residue of the RNA codon.

The $Gm^{3,5,10,11,13,14,26}$ haplotype is unique to Caucasoids. The only other haplotype that lacks Gm(1) and that occurs at polymorphic frequencies in any population is the $Gm^{2,17,21,26}$ haplotype of the Ainu, previously mentioned. We do not understand the significance of the restriction to these two races of haplotypes lacking Gm(1).

Examination of the data in Tables III-1 to III-24 will show that almost all Caucasoid populations have some admixture with other races. The admixture is primarily Negroid, but Mongoloid admixture is present in some populations, see Table III-13, for example, where the $Gm^{1,13}$ haplotype characteristic of Mongoloids is present.

Eighteen of the comparisons between the observed numbers and the expected numbers for the phenotypes derived from the Hardy–Weinberg (HW) equilibrium showed poor fits and interestingly, eleven were due to the Gm(2) allotype. In nine of these, Gm(1,2) was less frequent than expected and the Gm(1,2, 3,5,..) phenotype was more frequent than expected. We do not have an explanation for these data, which come from several different laboratories. We note that some data from the laboratories, included in the set of eleven showing poor fits to the HW distribution, show good fits to the HW equilibrium. We call attention, as a curiosity, to a sample from Cuba (Table III-2, p. 29) that gave a perfect fit to the HW distribution.

Many unusual phenotypes (and therefore unusual haplotypes) not due to admixture have been observed among the samples analysed in the studies listed in the tables. These are discussed in a separate section and will not be discussed here.

Khoisan

The Khoisan are composed of the San (Bushmen) and the Khoikhoi (Hottentots). Both of these populations have experienced considerable admixture. The San primarily with the Negroes and the Khoikhoi with Caucasoids and Negroes.

Three populations of Khoikhoi (Hottentots) have been tested for the Gm allotypes (Tables IV-1–3, pp. 66–8). All three populations show considerable evidence of Negroid admixture (the $Gm^{1,5,6,14}$ and $GM^{1,5,6}$ haplotypes) and two, the Topnaar and the Keetmanshoop populations, show evidence of Caucasoid admixture (the $Gm^{3,5,13,14}$ haplotype). The $Gm^{1,21}$ haplotype found among the Keetsmanshoop population suggests either Caucasoid or San admixture.

Only one of the three samples, that from the Sesfontein population, shows a satisfactory fit to the HW distribution and it is the one with no Caucasoid admixture, but it is also the smallest sample of the three.

The haplotype array of the Khoikhoi, as best we can tell from these data, is $Gm^{1,2,21}$, $Gm^{1,13}$, $Gm^{1,5,13,14}$, and $Gm^{1,5,14}$. More extensive testing (unpublished data) show these haplotypes to be $Gm^{1,2,17,21,26}$, $Gm^{1,10,11,13,15,17}$ (with or without Gm(16)), $Gm^{1,5,10,11,13,14,17,26}$, and $Gm^{1,5,10,11,14,17,26}$. The remaining haplotypes ($Gm^{1,21}$, $Gm^{1,5,6}$, $Gm^{1,5,6,14}$, and $Gm^{3,5,13,14}$) are probably due to admixture. The Khoikhoi are the only people to have $Gm^{1,2,21}$ without $Gm^{1,21}$.

Ten populations of San (Bushmen) have been tested (Tables IV-4 and 5, pp. 69–75). The data for only one population (Tsumkwe, p. 73) failed to fit the HW distribution. No evidence for Caucasoid or Khoikhoi admixture was present in any of the samples, but as stated above there was evidence for Negroid admixture. The data establish that the haplotype array among the San is $Gm^{1,21}$, $Gm^{1,13}$, $Gm^{1,5}$, $Gm^{1,5,13,14}$, and $Gm^{1,5,13,14,21}$. The last haplotype is unique to the San.

More extensive tests (unpublished data) have shown that the $Gm^{1,13}$ haplotype in the Khoisan is $Gm^{1,10,11,13,15,17}$ or $Gm^{1,10,11,13,15,16,17}$. The latter haplotype, but not the former, occurs among Mongoloid populations. The other haplotypes among the San are $Gm^{1,17,21,26}$, $Gm^{1,5,10,11,13,14,17,26}$, $Gm^{1,5,11,17,26}$, and $Gm^{1,5,10,11,13,14,17,21,26}$.

The haplotype arrays of the San and Khoikhoi differ in that the San have $Gm^{1,17,21,26}$, $Gm^{1,5,11,17,26}$, and $Gm^{1,5,10,11,13,14,17,21,26}$ which the Khoikhoi lack, and in that the Khoikhoi have $Gm^{1,2,17,21,26}$ which the San lack. The data indicate that these two very similar peoples have remained separate even though they at one time occupied, between them all of southern Africa (see Mourant et al. 1976 for review).

Lapps

The Lapps (Table V-1. p. 76) have a clearly Caucasoid array of Gm haplotypes, but they have, in addition, evidence of Mongoloid admixture ($Gm^{1,13}$ and $Gm^{1,3,5,13,14}$; tests for Gm(10,11,15,16, 17) have not been done). The Sevettijarvi Skolt Lapps have $Gm^{1,3,5,13,14,21}$ at polymorphic frequencies, but family data are needed to confirm the presence of this haplotype.

The origin of the Lapps is obscure (see Mourant et al. 1976 for review) as is their place in the classification of the human species. Their Gm types as well as the frequencies of alleles at blood group and enzyme loci indicate so many differences from other Caucasoids that it seems justified to treat them as a separate group.

Melanesians

Melanesians on New Guinea differ from those on the Solomon Islands in that they have the $Gm^{1,5,10,11,13,14,17,26}$ haplotype and in that speakers of Melanesian (MN) languages have a different array of haplotypes from speakers of non-Austronesian (NAN) languages (Tables VI-1–6). Giles, Ogan, and Steinberg (1965) showed, on the basis of tests for Gm(1,2,5,6), that the MN and NAN speakers in the Markham Valley differ from each other in that $Gm^{1,2}$ was essentially absent from the MN speakers and was present at polymorphic frequencies among the NAN speakers. Steinberg (1967) showed with tests for Gm(3), Gm(13), and Gm(14) that $Gm^{1,5}$ was $Gm^{1,3,5,13,14}$ or $Gm^{1,5,13,14}$, with the former haplotype being much more frequent among the MN speakers than among the NAN, and with the latter haplotype being about equally frequent in the two groups. Subsequent studies by others (Table VI-4, p. 84) confirmed this difference. The difference disappears among populations on Bougainville and on the Solomon Islands, where all populations are polymorphic for $Gm^{1,3,5,13,14}$, $Gm^{1,17,21}$, and $Gm^{1,2,17,21}$, which on more extensive testing become $Gm^{1,3,5,10,11,13,14,26}$, $Gm^{1,17,21,26}$, and $Gm^{1,2,17,21,26}$, respectively. The Lau on Malaita are unique among the Melanesians in that they are polymorphic for a $Gm^{1,2,5,13,14}$ haplotype. (It is probably $Gm^{1,2,5,10,11,13,14,17,26}$, but appropriate tests have not been done.)

Tests for Gm(23) (Table VI-6, p. 88) indicate that among both the MN and NAN speaking peoples on New Britain, the $Gm^{1,3,5,10,11,13,14}$ haplotype may occur with or without this allotype, but usually without it. The $Gm^{1,5,10,11,13,14,17}$ haplotype, which is much rarer among these people, does not occur without Gm(23), except for one population of NAN speakers (Mope Village) and one population of MN speakers (Nordup Village) (Table VI-6, p. 91). Only two populations of NAN speakers and one of MN speakers on New Guinea have been tested for Gm(23) (pp. 92 and 93). Gm (23) was not found in the $GM^{1,3,5,10,11,13,14}$ haplotype among the NAN speakers but it was found in the majority of such haplotypes among the MN speakers. The majority of the $Gm^{1,5,10,11,13,14,17}$ haplotypes among the NAN speakers and all of them among the MN speakers have Gm(23).

5

Micronesians

Relatively few populations of Micronesians have been tested for the Gm allotypes (Tables VII-1–3). The limited data combined with pedigree analyses indicate that the haplotypes of the Micronesians are $Gm^{1,3,5,13,14}$ and $Gm^{1,21}$ (probably $Gm^{1,3,5,10,11,13,14,26}$ and $Gm^{1,17,21,26}$, but appropriate tests have not been performed). The $Gm^{1,2,21}$ haplotype present in the populations listed in Table VII-2 (p. 95) was shown by analysis of extended pedigrees to have been introduced through white or Mongoloid admixture. In the same way, the $Gm^{1,5,6}$ and $Gm^{1,5,13,14}$ haplotypes in these populations were shown to have been introduced through black admixture (Morton, Lew, Hussels, and Little 1972).

The samples from the people on the Rongelap Atoll (Table VII-1, p. 94) were subsequently tested for Gm(3), Gm(13), and Gm(14) (Steinberg 1967). The Gm(1,5) samples proved to be Gm(1,3,5,13,14) and thus are consistent with the haplotype array listed above. The $Gm^{1,2,21}$ haplotype is much more frequent among the 48 samples from West Truk than among the samples from Kusai, Mokil, Pingelap, and Ponape. It is possible therefore that the presence of this haplotype among those on Truk is not due to admixture.

Mongoloids

Mongoloid populations have been tested for 27 different sets of allotypes (Tables VIII-1–27), but only one sample of Taiwan Aborigines, one sample of Japanese from Osaka, and one sample of Thais have been tested for Gm(23) (Tables VIII-24, 26, 27, pp. 133, 135, 136). In all three samples the $Gm^{1,3,5,10,11,13,(14)}$ haplotype was uniformly associated with Gm(23). One sample in the Thai series was Gm(1,2,17,21,23), indicating that Gm(23) may occur with $Gm^{1,2,17,21}$ in this population.

One Aborigine was Gm(1,3,17,21,23) providing evidence for the presence of a $Gm^{1,3,21,23}$ haplotype or for a $Gm^{1,3,21}$ haplotype. If the latter is correct, the phenotype requires a $Gm^{1,17,21,23}$ haplotype. In the former case only one unusual haplotype need be postulated; in the latter case two unusual haplotypes are required. Thus the former (i.e. a $Gm^{1,3,21,23}$ haplotype) seems more likely. Another possibility is a $Gm^{1,3,23}$ haplotype and this suggests that the haplotype fails to produce any $\gamma 3$ heavy chains.

The data for the Mongoloids (exclusive of Gm(23)) indicate that their haplotypes are $Gm^{1,17,21}$, $Gm^{1,2,17,21}$, $Gm^{1,10,11,13,15,16,17}$, and $Gm^{1,3,5,10,11,13,14}$ (Gm(26) occurs with each of these except $Gm^{1,10,11,13,15,16,17}$). Each of these haplotypes is present among the Mongoloid peoples of Asia and among Indians of Central America, but not among all the tribes so far tested (See the Tables on pp. 100, 105, 111, and 113). Most South American and North American Indian tribes appear to have only the $Gm^{1,17,21}$ and $Gm^{1,2,17,21}$ haplotypes. Exceptions are provided by the Athabascan Indians in Alaska, who have the entire array of haplotypes, and some South American tribes (notably those on Suriname and French Guiana, pp. 131 and 132) who appear to have the $Gm^{1,10,11,13,15,16,17}$ haplotype. All Eskimo tribes seem to have $Gm^{1,17,21}$, $Gm^{1,2,17,21}$, $Gm^{1,13,15,16,17}$ (pp. 108, 114, 117 and 119), but only some have $Gm^{1,3,5,10,11,13,14}$. Thus the situation is similar to that among the Amerindians.

Negroids

The data in Tables IX-1–11 plus data from this laboratory not included in this monograph establish that Negroids have the haplotypes $Gm^{1,5,10,11,13,14,17,26}$, $Gm^{1,5,10,11,14,17,26}$, $Gm^{1,5,6,11,17,24,26}$, and $Gm^{1,5,6,10,11,14,17,26}$. Unfortunately Negroids have not been tested for Gm(23). The $Gm^{1,5,10,11,14,17,26}$ haplotype is the least common and has been found only in a few tribes (Table IX-9, p. 146).

Many of the southern African tribes have a significant amount of San admixture as evidenced by the presence of the $Gm^{1,13}$ (this is $Gm^{1,10,11,13,15,17}$ with or without Gm(16) when adequate tests have been performed).

The data for the Surinam populations (Table IX-8, p. 144) do not fit the Hardy–Weinberg distribution when tests for Gm(2) are included. Gm(2) in the Paramaribo Region population is due exclusively to the $Gm^{1,2}$ haplotype (i.e. $Gm^{1,2,17,21}$ haplotype); it is due to this haplotype and to the $Gm^{1,2,5,11,13}$ haplotype in the non-Paramaribo Region. The $Gm^{1,2,17,21}$ haplotype and the $Gm^{1,17,21}$ haplotype are due to admixture with Caucasoids or Indians. The $Gm^{3,5,11,13}$ haplotype is of Caucasoid origin. It is not apparent why haplotypes containing the Gm(2) antigen should cause a poor fit to the Hardy–Weinberg distribution while other haplotypes due to admixture fit the HW distribution.

The $Gm^{1,2,5,11,13}$ (really $Gm^{1,2,5,10,11,13,14,26}$) haplotype is not polymorphic among these people, nor among other Africans, but it is polymorphic among the Lau on Malaita (Table VI-3, p. 82).

Polynesians

So far as we are aware, only 94 samples from Hawaiians of mixed ancestry have been tested for Gm antigens. Unfortunately, the samples were tested for only Gm(1,2,5,6). The haplotypes found: $Gm^{1,5}$, $Gm^{1,2}$, and Gm^{1}, probably represent $Gm^{1,3,5,10,11,13,14,26}$, $Gm^{1,2,17,21,26}$, and $Gm^{1,17,21,26}$. If this is the correct haplotype array for Polynesians, it is identical with that of Melanesians on Bougainville and the Solomon Islands and would represent the first instance of two races having the same haplotype array.

Negritos

Forty-eight serum samples from Negritos in Malaysia (Table XI-3, p. 159) and a larger number from each of the three tribes in the Philippines (Table XI-6, p. 163) have been tested for Gm antigens. It is clear that Negritos have haplotypes $Gm^{1,17,21}$, and $Gm^{1,3,5,11,13,14}$ which, as noted above, constitute the haplotype array of the few Polynesians who have been tested and of the Melanesians not on New Guinea. There is evidence for the presence of the $Gm^{1,5,11,13,14,17}$ haplotype and the unusual $Gm^{1,5,11,13,14,15,17}$ haplotype among these people. The latter haplotype was observed in two of the 127 samples from Zambales on Luzon and in none of the samples among the other two tribes from the Philippines. The $Gm^{1,5,11,13,14,17}$ haplotype was present in all three tribes but at low frequencies (≤ 3 per cent) which raises the question of possible admixture.

3 Unusual phenotypes (haplotypes)

Caucasoids

A list of unusual phenotypes among Caucasoids, not explicable by racial admixture, is presented in Table 3.

The Gm(−) phenotype (No. 1) has been observed among the Hutterites (Steinberg, Muir, and McIntire 1968). Extensive family studies established the presence of a Gm^- haplotype that lacks all allotypes on the $\gamma 1$ and $\gamma 3$ chains. The haplotype leads to the production of a hybrid molecule with the N-terminal half being $\gamma 3$ and the remainder $\gamma 1$ (Kunkel et al. 1969; Steinberg, Terry, and Morrell 1970). There is reason to believe that the

hinge region is $\gamma 3$ (Werner and Steinberg 1974; and unpublished data of Steinberg, Frangione, and Franklin). It is not known if the Gm(−) phenotype in Table 3 is the same as that among the Hutterites. It very likely is not, because three of the 500 samples from unrelated blood donors or people involved in paternity tests were reported to be Gm(−); i.e. homozygous for a Gm^- haplotype. It is therefore likely that some technical problem, rather than an unusual haplotype, is the explanation for the Gm(−) phenotype. The authors did not discuss their results.

The Gm(2,5) and the Gm(2,3,5) phenotypes (Nos. 2 and 5, respectively) may be explained by the $Gm^{2,5}$ haplotype which

Table 3 Unusual Gm phenotypes among Caucasoids not explicable by racial admixture

	Phenotype	Tested for	Table	Page	Allotype expected to be Present	Absent
(1)	blank	1,2,5	III-2	25	at least one	
(2)	2,5		III-2	27, 29	1	
	2,5	1,2,5,6	III-6	36	1	
(3)	1,3	1,3,5	III-4	31	5	or 3
	1,3	1,2,3,5	III-5	32	5	or 3
	1,3		III-5	34	5	or 3
	1,3	1,2,3,5,10	III-7	38	5,10	or 3
	1,3	1,2,3,5,10,11	III-23	64	5,10,11	or 3
(4)	1,2,3	1,2,3,5,10	III-7	38	5,10	or 3
(5)	2,3,5	1,2,3,5	III-5	32	1	
(6)	5,10	1,2,3,5,10	III-7	38	3	
(7)	1,2,3,5		III-7	38	10	
(8)	1,2,3,5,10,11	1,2,3,5,10,11,21	III-12	42	21	
(9)	1,3,21	1,2,3,5,6,13,14,21	III-13	45, 46	5,13,14	or 3
(10)	1,3,13,21		III-13	46	5,14	or 3
(11)	1,2,3,5,10,11,17	1,2,3,5,10,11,17,21	III-14	47	21	
(12)	3,5,10,11,21		III-14	47		21
(13)	1,2,3,11,17,21		III-14	47	5,10	or 3,11
(14)	1,3,17,21		III-14	47		3
	1,3,17,21	1,2,3,5,6,10,11,13,14,17,21	III-15	49		3
	1,3,17,21	1,2,3,5,6,10,11,13,15,16,17,21,24	III-16	50		3
	1,3,17,21	1,2,3,5,6,10,11,13,15,16,17,21,23,24	III-17	57		3
(15)	3,5,10,11,17	1,2,3,5,10,11,17,21	III-14	47		17
(16)	1,2,3,5,10,11,13,14,17	1,2,3,5,6,10,11,13,14,17,21	III-15	49	21	or 2
(17)	1,3,5,6,10,11,13,14,17,21		III-15	49		6 or 21
(18)	1,3,5,6,10,11,14,17		III-15	49	13	6
(19)	1,2,3,17,21	1,2,3,5,6,11,13,15,16,17,21,24	III-16	50		3
(20)	1,2,3,5,11,13,17		III-16	50	21	or 2
(21)	3,5,6,11,13		III-16	50	10	and 6
(22)	3,5,10,11,13,15,23,24	1,2,3,5,6,10,11,13,15,16,17,21,23,24	III-17	52,53,54,55,56		15,24
(23)	1,3,5,10,11,13,15,17,21,23,24		III-17	52,53,54		15,24
(24)	1,3,5,10,11,13,15,17,23,24		III-17	56		15,24
(25)	3,5,10,11,13,21,23		III-17	57		21
(26)	1,3,5,11,17,21,23,24		III-17	57	10,13	and 24
(27)	3,5,10,11,13,23,24		III-17	57		24
(28)	1,3,5,10,11,13,15,17,21,23		III-17	57		15
(29)	1,2,3,5,10,11,13,17,23		III-17	57	21	
(30)	1,5,6,10,11,13,17,21,23		III-17	57		6 or 13
(31)	1,2,3,5,10,11,13,14,17,23	1,2,3,5,10,11,13,14,17,21,23	III-21	62	21	

has been established by family studies involving samples tested for Gm(1,2,5) only (Henningsen and Neilsen 1961; and many others).

Phenotypes Gm(5,10) and Gm(1,2,3,5) (Nos. 6 and 7) were reported in the course of studies designed to shed information on Gm(4) (now Gm(3)) and on Gm(18). The investigators did not comment on these unusual phenotypes other than to note them. The Gm(1,2,3,5,10,11) phenotype (No. 8) probably involves a $Gm^{1,2,5,10,11}$ haplotype, as does phenotype (No. 11). Gm(17) should be added to the haplotype in the latter case.

The Gm(1,3,17,21) phenotype (No. 14) has been observed in several Caucasoid populations (Table 3). It has been shown to have a $Gm^{1,3,17,21}$ haplotype among the Hutterites (Steinberg et al. 1968; Steinberg et al. 1970) and in some isolated families (Natvig, Kunkel, and Litwin 1967; Steinberg et al. 1970); a Gm^3 haplotype in a large kindred (Lefranc, Rivat, Rivat, Loiselet, and Ropartz 1976) and among Jews from Cochin, India (Steinberg and Cook 1977; Steinberg et al. unpublished data); and a $Gm^{1,3,21}$ haplotype among Parsi and Irani (Steinberg, Undevia, and Tepfenhart 1973). The $Gm^{1,3,17,21}$, $Gm^{1,3,21}$, and Gm^3 haplotypes have been confirmed by family data. The Gm(1,3), Gm(1,2,3), Gm(1,3,21), Gm(1,3,13,21), and Gm(1, 2,3,17,21) phenotypes (Nos. 3, 4, 9, 10, 19, respectively) may also be explained by one or more of the above haplotypes. Tests for more allotypes and family data are needed for a conclusion to be drawn concerning which of the haplotypes is involved in each of these phenotypes.

The $Gm^{1,3,17,21}$ haplotype is probably due to a duplication since Gm(3) and Gm(17) appear to involve amino acid substitutions at residue 214 (Eu numbering), Arg for Gm(3) and Lys for Gm(17) (Edelman, Cunningham, Gall, Gottlieb, Rattishauser, and Waxdal 1969). The $Gm^{1,3,21}$ haplotype could have been derived from the common $Gm^{1,17,21}$ haplotype by a mutation involving a single nucleotide.

The Gm^3 haplotype requires a change leading to the failure to produce any detectable $\gamma3$ chains (Lefranc et al. 1976; Steinberg and Cook 1977; Steinberg et al. unpublished data). It could be due to a deficiency, to a chain terminating mutation or to any one of several changes having to do with the association of the V (variable) region with the C (constant) region, or with chain initiation or other aspects of translation, or with transcription.

In the absence of family data, several haplotypes may be suggested to account for the Gm(3,5,10,11,21) and Gm(1,2,3, 11,17,21) phenotypes (Nos. 12 and 13). We shall not speculate about them.

The Gm(3,5,10,11,17) phenotype (No. 15) suggests the presence of a Gm^{17} haplotype (other haplotypes are also possible; for example $Gm^{3,5,10,11,17}$, $Gm^{5,10,11,17}$, etc.). Once again, family data are required. Eight out of 167 samples from Persian Jews (Cohen, T., Steinberg, A. G., Levene, C., unpublished) had the phenotype Gm(3,5,13,14,17) when tested for Gm(1,2,3,5,6,13, 14,17,21). The population data gave a satisfactory fit to the Hardy–Weinberg distribution with each of the following haplotypes: Gm^{17}, $Gm^{5,13,14,17}$, and $Gm^{3,5,13,14,17}$, the only three tried. No choice may be made in the absence of the family data, but we are inclined to believe that the second haplotype is the most likely, because it can arise from the common haplotype $Gm^{3,5,13,14}$, by a mutation involving a single nucleotide, leading to the replacement of Gm(3) by Gm(17).

Phenotypes 22–24, observed among Sardinians, are concerned with the anomalous presence of Gm(15) and Gm(24). They suggest the presence of a $Gm^{3,5,10,11,13,15,23,24}$ haplotype, but once again we must state that family data are required. We have also

detected the same anomalous presence of Gm(24) in samples from Sardinians, kindly sent to us by Dr Ropartz. We note, however, that tests with several reagent systems, that give concordant results in tests for Gm(24) on samples from Negroids, give discordant results when used on the Sardinian samples (unpublished data). We are inclined to think that the anomalous allotype is not Gm(24) but some still unidentified allotype. This, of course, still leaves the anomalous presence of Gm(15) unexplained.

Phenotypes Nos. 16, 20, and 29 (Gm(1,2,3,5,10,11,13,14,17), Gm(1,2,3,5,11,13,17), and Gm(1,2,3,5,10,11,13,17,23), respectively; phenotype 20 is for a sample that was not tested for Gm(10)) may be explained by assuming the presence of the $Gm^{1,2,5,10,11,13,17}$ haplotype with or without Gm(23). Such a haplotype has on occasion been observed in blacks and at polymorphic frequency in a Melanesian population (Table VI-3, pp. 82, 83). This haplotype may also explain phenotype 31 (Gm(1,2,3,5,10,11,13,14,17,23)).

Phenotypes Gm(1,3,4,6,10,11,13,14,17,21), Gm(1,3,5,6,10, 11,14,17), and Gm(3,5,6,11,13) (Nos, 17, 18, and 21) concern the unexpected presence of Gm(6). Once again family data are required to determine the haplotypes involved. We wonder if the Gm(6) recorded in these phenotypes may not be related to the unidentified allotype mentioned in the discussion of the Sardinian samples.

The Gm(3,5,10,11,13,21,23) phenotype (No. 25) suggests the presence of a $Gm^{3,21}$ haplotype, but other haplotypes such as Gm^{21} (i.e. one producing no $\gamma1$ chains), $Gm^{3,5,10,11,13,21,23}$, etc., are possible. Family data are needed to identify the haplotype.

Phenotype No. 28 (Gm(1,3,5,10,11,13,15,17,21,23)) may be explained by assuming a $Gm^{3,5,10,11,13,15,23}$ or a $Gm^{1,13,15,17,21}$ haplotype, but, as usual, family data are needed. Phenotype No. 30 (Gm(1,5,6,10,11,13,17,21,23)) suggests a haplotype in which Gm(6) and Gm(13) are present simultaneously, e.g. $Gm^{1,5,6,10,11,13,17,23}$. Family data are needed to confirm this.

Mongoloids

The unusual phenotypes observed among Mongoloids are listed in Table 4. The $Gm^{1,3}$ or $Gm^{1,3,21}$ haplotype occurs among Mongoloids (phenotypes 1,2,6,22,28,29,31, and 32; Table 4), as well as among Caucasoids. (Phenotype 32 is included because of the data for the entire sample.) This is not surprising since $Gm^{1,17,21}$ is common among Mongoloids and, as indicated earlier, it can give rise to the $Gm^{1,3,21}$ haplotype by a simple mutation. Phenotypes 31 and 32 may be explained by the presence of a $Gm^{1,2,21}$ haplotype which appears to be present in the Thai population from which these samples came, but, as usual, family studies are required. Phenotypes 23 and 24 may be explained by a $Gm^{1,3,13,16}$ haplotype rather than by a $Gm^{1,3}$ haplotype. The $Gm^{1,3,13,16}$ haplotype may be derived from the $Gm^{1,13,16,17}$ haplotype by a simple mutation of Gm(17) to Gm(3).

Phenotype 3 (Gm(1,3,10)) indicates a $Gm^{1,3,10}$ haplotype, i.e. one lacking Gm(5), while phenotype 4 (Gm(1,3,5)) indicates a $Gm^{1,3,5}$ haplotype, i.e. one lacking Gm(10,11). Phenotypes 5 and 8 (Gm(1,5,10,17,21) and Gm(1,3,5,10,17,21), respectively) lack Gm(14). (The former also lacks Gm(3).) Phenotype 7 (Gm(1,3,14,17,21)) on the other hand unexpectedly has Gm(14) which suggests a $Gm^{1,3,14}$ haplotype. Phenotype 9 (Gm(1,10,17, 21)) surprisingly has Gm(10).

Phenotypes 10,11,12,13,15,16,17,18,19, and 20 all involve the anomalous presence of Gm(16) in an array of haplotypes

Table 4 Unusual Gm phenotypes among Mongoloids not explicable by racial admixture

	Phenotype	Tested for	Table	Page	Allotype expected to be Present	Absent
(1)	1,3	1,2,3,5	VIII-4	100	5	or 3
(2)	1,2,3	1,2,3,5,10	VIII-8	106	5,10	or 3
(3)	1,3,10		VIII-8	106	5	
(4)	1,3,5	1,2,3,5,10,11	VIII-9	107	10,11	
(5)	1,5,10,17,21	1,2,3,5,10,14,17,21	VIII-16	119	3,14	
(6)	1,2,3,17,21		VIII-16	119		3
(7)	1,3,14,17,21		VIII-16	119	5,10	or 3,14
(8)	1,3,5,10,17,21		VIII-16	119	14	
(9)	1,10,17,21		VIII-16	119		10
(10)	1,5,11,13,16,21	1,2,3,5,6,11,13,16,21	VIII-18	122		5 or 6
(11)	1,16,21		VIII-18	122		16
(12)	1,2,16,21		VIII-18	122		16
(13)	1,2,3,5,11,13,16,21		VIII-18	122		16
(14)	1,2,11,13,16		VIII-18	122	21	or 2
(15)	1,16		VIII-18	122	21	and 16
(16)	1,3,5,13,16,21	1,2,3,5,6,13,16,21,24	VIII-20	125		16 or 21
(17)	1,2,3,5,13,16,21		VIII-20	125		3 or 16
(18)	1,2,5,13,16,21		VIII-20	125		5 or 16
(19)	1,5,13,16,21		VIII-20	125		5 or 16
(20)	1,3,5,11,13,16,21	1,2,3,5,6,11,13,16,21,24	VIII-21	126		16
(21)	5,11,13		VIII-21	126	1,3	
(22)	1,2,3,21		VIII-21	126		3
(23)	1,2,3,13,16,21		VIII-21	126	11	3
(24)	1,3,13,16		VIII-21	126	11	3
(25)	1,2,3,5,11,13,16		VIII-21	126		2
(26)	1,2,3,5,11,13		VIII-21	126,128	21	or 2
(27	1,2		VIII-21	126	21	
(28)	1,3,17,21,23	1,2,3,5,11,13,15,16,17,21,23	VIII-24	133		3
(29)	1,3,11,13,15,16,17,21,23	1,2,3,5,6,11,13,15,16,17,21,23,24	VIII-26	135		3
(30)	1,2,3,5,10,11,13,17,23	1,2,3,5,6,10,11,13,15,16,17,21,23,24	VIII-27	136	21	or 2
(31)	1,3,5,10,11,13,21,23		VIII-27	136	17	or 21
(32)	1,3,5,10,11,13,17,21		VIII-27	136	23	or 3

that offers no consistent pattern. However, it should be noted that a $Gm^{1,16,21}$ haplotype could explain phenotypes 10,11,12, 16, and 19. Since all these samples were examined in the same laboratory we wonder if there is something unusual about the anti-Gm(16) antibody used for these analyses.

Phenotype 14 (Gm(1,2,11,13,16)) and phenotype 27 (Gm(1,2)) suggest a $Gm^{1,2}$ haplotype, i.e. one failing to produce a γ3 chain. Phenotype 27 would represent homozygosity for the haplotype. Phenotype 21 (Gm(5,11,13)), on the other hand, suggests homozygosis for a haplotype that fails to produce a γ1 chain.

Phenotypes 25, 26, and 30 all show the unexpected presence of Gm(2) which may be explained by assuming the presence of a $Gm^{1,2,3,5,11,13}$ haplotype.

Negroids

The unusual phenotypes observed among Negroids are listed in Table 5. They are surprisingly few; possibly because fewer population studies have been done on Negroids than on Caucasoids or on Mongoloids, but possibly also because there is less variation among the haplotypes that are common among Negroids.

Phenotypes No. 1, 4, 5 (Gm(5,6), Gm(5,6,13,14), and Gm(5,13,14), respectively) involve the unexpected absence of

Table 5 Unusual Gm phenotypes among Negroids not explicable by racial admixture

	Phenotype	Tested for	Table	Page	Allotype expected to be Present	Absent
(1)	5,6	1,2,5,6	IX-3	140	1	
(2)	1,5	1,2,3,5,10	IX-5	142	10	or 5
	1,5	1,2,3,5,6,13,14	IX-9	148	6 or 13,14	or 5
[a](3)	1,2,5,6,11,13	1,2,3,5,6,11,13	IX-8	144		2
[b](4)	5,6,13,14	1,2,3,5,6,13,14	IX-9	148	1	
[c](5)	5,13,14		IX-9	148	1	
[a](6)	1,2,5,13,14		IX-9	148,150,152	21	or 2

[a] Subsequently tested for Gm(21) and found to be negative.
[b] H-chain concentrations normal.
[c] Absent γ1 and elevated γ3 shown by Terry (personal communication).

Gm(1). These phenotypes could result if the donors failed to produce a $\gamma 1$ heavy chain or if they produced one without allotypes. The donor of the sample with phenotype 5 (Gm(5,13, 14)) was shown by Dr W. D. Terry (personal communication) to lack the $\gamma 1$ heavy chain and to have an increased amount of the $\gamma 3$ chain.

The Gm(1,5) phenotype (No. 2) suggests an unusual $\gamma 3$ chain, i.e. one lacking the usual array of allotypes.

Phenotypes 3 and 6 (Gm(1,2,5,6,11,13) and Gm(1,2,5,13, 14)) concern the unexpected presence of Gm(2). They may be explained by the presence of $Gm^{1,2,5,13,14}$ haplotype, which seems to occur rarely among Negroids. It has been observed at polymorphic frequencies among a Melanesian tribe (the Lau) on the Island of Malaita (Table VI-3, p. 82).

Discussion

The arrays of unusual phenotypes that are listed in Table 3, 4, and 5, and the unusual haplotypes required to explain them, suggest that virtually any combination of allotypes may occur in a haplotype. If those haplotypes which require duplications are excluded from consideration, we are confronted with the question of why the unusual haplotypes are unusual. This question is the complement of one arising from a consideration of the common haplotypes, e.g. why are common haplotypes common? More specifically, why do certain allotypes which are common in all races occur in haplotypes in some races but not in other races? For example, why do Gm(1) and Gm(3), or Gm(1) and Gm(5) not occur in a haplotype among Caucasoids, among whom these allotypes are common? Haplotypes with these combinations of allotypes are common in other races. We could raise a series of similar questions, but we see no point in doing so. We no more have answers to these questions than we have answers to the questions, 'Why do only Caucasoids and Ainu have haplotypes lacking Gm(1)?' or 'Why do the haplotype arrays differ among the various races?'

As stated earlier, Gm(1) has a frequency of 100 per cent in all races except the Caucasoid and the Ainu. Similarly, Gm(17) has a frequency of 100 per cent among the Ainu, Negroids, Australian Aborigines, and the Khoisan. Negroids are the only people who do not have Gm(21) and they are the only people who have Gm(6) and Gm(24) at polymorphic frequencies. In a similar manner, Gm(15) and Gm(16) are limited to Mongoloids and the Khoisan.

The extraordinary linkage disequilibrium demonstrated by the Gm haplotypes, far greater than any shown by the HLA haplotypes, remains unexplained. It is astonishing that in Caucasoids the frequencies of the $\gamma 1$ allotype Gm(3) and of the $\gamma 3$ allotypes Gm(5), Gm(10), Gm(11), Gm(13), Gm(14), and Gm(26) are identical, and that the $\gamma 1$ allotypes Gm(1) and Gm(17) have the same frequency as the $\gamma 3$ allotype Gm(21). It is equally surprising that Gm(15) and Gm(16) always occur together among Mongoloids, while this is not true of their occurrence among the Khoisan. Such patterns occur for many other combinations of allotypes, but we see no reason to labour the point.

The regularity of the distributions of the allotypes and haplotypes among the races and the existence of clines of the haplotypes within races (see maps) strongly suggests that selection has played a major role in shaping these distributions. Surprisingly, because these allotypes are carried by the immunoglobulins, we have no idea what force or forces of selection are in operation.

It has been suggested many times that the haplotypes might influence the effectiveness of antibodies against various pathogens. Alternatively, the haplotypes might affect the several functions associated with the constant region of the chains, but once again we have no evidence for this suggestion. We urge immunologists with skills in these areas to determine if there is any merit in our suggestion.

References cited in text

ALLISON, A. C. (1961). Abnormal haemoglobin and erythrocyte enzyme-deficiency traits. In *Genetical variation in human populations* (ed. G. A. Harrison), pp. 16–40. Pergamon Press New York.

BOYD, W. C. (1939). Blood groups. *Tabul. biol.* **ii**, 113–240.

EDELMAN, G. M., CUNNINGHAM, B. A, GALL, W. E., GOTTLIEB, P. D., RATTISHAUSER, U., and WAXDAL, M. J. (1969). The covalent structure of an entire γG immunoglobulin molecule. *Proc. natn. Acad. Sci. U.S.A.* **63**, 78–85.

FRIEDLAENDER, J. S. (1975). *Patterns of human variation.* Harvard University Press, Cambridge.

—— and STEINBERG, A. G. (1970). Anthropological significance of gamma globulin (Gm and Inv) antigens in Bougainville Island, Melanesia. *Nature, Lond.* **228**, 59–61.

GIBLETT, E. R. (1969). *Genetic markers in human blood.* Blackwell, Oxford.

GILES, E., OGAN, E., and STEINBERG, A. G. (1965). Gamma-globulin factors (Gm and Inv) in New Guinea: Anthropological significance. *Science, Wash.* **150**, 1158–60.

GOLD, E. R. and FUDENBERG, H. H. (1967). Chromic chloride: a coupling reagent for passive hemagglutination reactions. *J. Immun.* **99**, 859–66.

GRUBB, R. (1956). Agglutination of erythrocytes coated with "incomplete" anti-Rh by certain rheumatoid arthritic sera and some other sera. The existence of human serum groups. *Acta path. microb. scand.* **39**, 195–7.

—— (1961). Hereditary gamma globulin groups in man. *Am. J. hum. Genet.* **13**, 171–4.

—— (1970). *The genetic markers of human immunoglobulins.* Springer-Verlag, New York.

—— and LAURELL, A. B-. (1956). Hereditary serological human serum groups. *Acta path. microbiol. scand.* **39**, 390–8.

HENNINGSEN, K. and NIELSEN, J. C. (1961). A rare phenotype within the Gm system. *Nature, Lond.* **192**, 476.

HIRSCHFELD, L. and HIRSCHFELD, H. (1919). Serological differences between the blood of different races. The result of researches on the Macedonian front. *Lancet* **ii**, 675–79.

JOHNSON, W. E., KOHN, P. H., and STEINBERG, A. G. (1977a). Population genetics of the human allotypes Gm, Inv, and A2m. *Clin. Immunobiol, and Immunopathol.* **7**, 97–113.

——, ——, —— (1977b). Gm and Km(Inv) frequencies in two Roumanian populations. *Am. J. hum. Genet.* **39**, 199–211.

KUNKEL, H. G., NATVIG, J. B., and JOSLIN, F. G. (1969). A "Lepore" type of hybrid γ-globulin. *Proc. natn. Acad. Sci. U.S.A.* **62**, 144–9.

——, SMITH, W. K., JOSLIN, F. G., NATVIG, J. B., and LITWIN, S. D. (1969). Genetic marker of the γA2 subgroup of γA immunoglobulins. *Nature, Lond.* **223**, 1247–8.

KURCZYNSKI, T. W. and STEINBERG, A. G. (1967). A general program for maximum likelihood estimation of gene frequencies. *Am. J. hum. Genet.* **19**, 178–9.

LEFRANC, G., RIVAT, L., RIVAT, C., LOISELET, J., and ROPARTZ, C. (1976). Evidence for "Deleted " or "Salent" gene homozygous at the locus coding for the constant region of the γ3 chain. *Am. J. hum. Genet.* **28**, 51–61.

van LOGHEM, E. and MARTENSSON, L. (1968). Gm(x) in Negroes. *Vox Sang.* **14**, 258–63.

——, WANG, A. C., and SHUSTER, J. (1973). A new genetic marker of human immunoglobulins determined by an allele at the α2 locus. *Vox Sang.* **24**, 481–8.

MAYR, E. (1963). *Animal species and evolution.* Harvard University Press, Cambridge, Mass.

McMICHAEL, M. and McDEVITT, H. (1977). The association between the HLA system and disease. *Prog. med. Genet.* **2**n.s., 39–100.

MENOZZI, P., PIAZZA A., and CAVALLI-SFORZA, L. (1978). Synthetic maps of human gene frequencies in Europeans. *Science Wash.* **201**, 786–94.

MILSTEIN, C. P., STEINBERG, A. G., McLAUGHLIN, C. L., and SOLOMON, E. (1974). Amino acid sequence change associated with genetic marker Inv(2) of human immunoglobulin. *Nature, Lond.* **248**, 160–1.

MORTON, N. E., LEW, R., HUSSELS, I. E., and LITTLE, G. F. (1972). Pingelap and Mokil Atolls: Historical genetics. *Am. J. hum. Genet.* **24**, 277–89.

MOURANT, A. E. (1954). *The distribution of the human blood groups.* Charles C. Thomas, Springfield, Illinois.

——, KOPEĆ, A. C., and DOMANIEWSKA-SOBCZAK, K. (1976). *The distribution of the human blood groups and other polymorphisms*, (2nd. edn.) Oxford University Press.

NATVIG, J. B. and KUNKEL, H. G. (1973). Human immunoglobulins: classes, subclasses, genetic variants, and idiotypes. *Adv. Immunol.* **16**, 1–59.

——, KUNKEL, H. G., and LITWIN, S. D. (1967). Genetic markers of the heavy chain subgroups of human γG globulin. *Cold Spring Harb. Symp. quant. Biol.* **32**, 173–80.

OMOTO, K. (1972). Polymorphisms and genetic affinities of the Ainu of Hokkaido. *Hum. Biol. Oceania* **1**, 278–88.

OUDIN, J. (1966). Genetic regulation of immunoglobulin synthesis. *J. cell comp. Physiol.* Suppl 1. **67**, 77–108.

RENFREW, C. (1973). *Before civilization.* Alfred A. Knopf, New York.

ROPARTZ, C., LENOIR, J., HEMET, Y., and RIVAT, L. (1960). Possible origins of the anti-Gm sera. *Nature, Lond.* **188**, 1120–1.

——, ——, and RIVAT, L. (1961). A new inheritable property of human sera: the InV factor. *Nature, Lond.* **189**, 586.

——, ROUSSEAU, P. Y-., RIVAT, L., BAITSCH, H., RITTER, H., PINKERTON, F. J., and MERMOD, L. E. (1964). Les groupes de γ-globulines Gm et Inv parmi la population d'Honolulu (Hawaii). *Acta genet. Basel* **14**, 25–35.

SCHANFIELD, M. S. (1971). Population studies on the Gm and Inv antigens in Asia and Oceania. Ph.D. Thesis, library of University of Michigan.

——, HERZOG, P., and FUNDENBERG, H. H. (1975). Immunoglobulin allotypes of European populations. II. Gm, Am, and Km(Inv) allotypic markers in Czechoslovakians. *Hum. Hered.* **25**, 382–92.

SIMMONS, R. T., GRAYDON, J. J., SEMPLE, N. M., and KODAMA, S. (1953). A collaborative genetical survey in Ainu: Hidaka, Island of Hokkaido. *Am. J. phys. Anthrop.* **11**, 47–82.

STEINBERG, A. G. (1967). Genetic variations in human immunoglobulins: The Gm and Inv types. In *Advances in Immunogenetics* (ed. T. J. Greenwalt), pp. 75–98. Lippincott Co., Philadelphia.

——, (1969). Globulin polymorphisms in man. *A. Rev. Genet.* **3**, 25–52.

——, GILES, B. D., and STAUFFER, R. (1960a). A Gm-like factor present in Negroes and rare or absent in whites: Its relation to Gmᵃ and Gmˣ. *Am. J. hum. Genet.* **12**, 44–51.

——, STAUFFER, R., and FUDENBERG, H. (1960b). Distribution of Gmᵃ and Gm-like among Japanese, Djuka Negroes, and Oyana and Carib Indians. *Nature, Lond.* **185**, 324–5.

——, WILSON, J. A., and LANSET, S. (1962). A new human gamma globulin factor determined by an allele at the Inv locus. *Vox Sang.* **7**, 151–6.

——, and MATSUMOTO, H. (1964). Studies on the Gm, Inv, Hp, and Tf serum factors of Japanese populations and families. *Hum. Biol.* **36**, 77–85.

——, MUIR, W. A., and McINTIRE, S. A. (1968). Two unusual Gm alleles: Their implications for the genetics of the Gm antigens. *Am. J. hum. Genet.* **20**, 258–78.

——, and KIRK, R. L. (1970). Gm and Inv types of Aborigines in the Northern Territory of Australia. *Archaeol. phys. Anthrop. Oceania* **V**, 163–72.

——, TERRY, W. D., and MORRELL, A. R. (1970). Human allotypes and genetic dogma. In *Protides of biological fluids.* (ed. J. Peeters), Ch. 17, pp. 111–16. Pergamon Press, Oxford.

——, DAMON, A., and BLOOM, J. (1972). Gammaglobulin allotypes of Melanesians from Malaita and Bougainville, Solomon Islands. *Am. J. phys. Anthrop*. **36**, 77–84.

——, UNDEVIA, J. V., and TEPFENHART, M.A. (1973). Gm and Inv studies of Parsi and Irani in India; Report of a new polymorphic haplotype, $Gm^{1,3,21}$. *Am. J. hum. Genet*. **25**, 302–9.

——, MILSTEIN, C. P., McLAUGHLIN, C. L., and SOLOMON, A. (1974). Structural studies of an Inv(1,2) kappa light chain. *Immunogenet*. **1**, 108–17.

——, and COOK, C. E. (1977). Failure of anti-γ3 antibodies to detect some γ3 chains by an agglutination inhibition test. *J. immunol. Methods* **17**, 147–52.

——, LEVINE, C., YODFAT, Y., FIDEL, J., BRAUTBAR, C., and COHEN, T. Genetic studies on Jewish communities in Israel. Gm and Inv data for the Cochin Jews: Polymorphism for Gm^3 and for $Gm^{1,17,21}$ without Gm(26). (In preparation.)

TERRY, W. D., FAHEY, J. L., and STEINBERG, A. G. (1965). Gm and Inv factors in subclasses of human IgG. *J. exp. Med*. **122**, 1087–1102.

VYAS, G. N. and FUDENBERG, H. H. (1969). Am(1), the first genetic marker of human immunoglobulin A. *Proc. natn. Acad. Sci. U.S.A*. **64**, 1211–16.

WERNER, B. G. and STEINBERG, A. G. (1974). Structural studies of a human hybrid immunoglobulin. *Immunogenet*. **1**, 254–71.

WORLD HEALTH ORGANIZATION (1965). Notation for genetic factors of human immunoglobulin. *Bull. Wld. Hlth. Org*. **33**, 721–4.

TABLES

4   Discussion of the tables

Selection of data for analysis

There is a vast amount of published data for population samples tested for only Gm(1), or for Gm(1) and Gm(2), or for Gm(1) and Gm(5). While we have compiled these data, they have not been included in this monograph. Such data are useful only for Caucasoid populations, but data for many more completely tested samples from Caucasiods are available; hence for all populations only samples tested for at least three allotypes have been included.

We have attempted to analyse all data published through 1976. These have been supplemented by more recently published data or by unpublished data from this laboratory when they supply information for regions of the world from which samples have not been previously collected.

All the data were analysed or reanalysed by means of the computer program MAXIM (Kurczynski and Steinberg 1967) as modified for this study. The printout was modified to provide tables that list the data for a series of populations in sequence, and the estimation of χ^2 was modified so that the values for classes with expectancies of less than one are accumulated until an expected value ≥ 1 is attained. This is done by adding the lowest expectancy to the next lowest and their sum to the next lowest, etc., until the total equals or exceeds one. The number of degrees of freedom is estimated by the program by subtracting the number of haplotypes used in the analysis from the number of comparisons with expected values ≥ 1.

Arrangement and numbering of the tables

The tables provide the χ^2 values and the degrees of freedom, but there is no indication of whether the difference between the observed and expected values is significant. Table 6 enables the reader to interpret the χ^2 values.

The data from some populations may be explained by using two or more different arrays of haplotypes. In such cases the expected values derived for the phenotype frequencies for each of the haplotype arrays are listed in sequence under the observed values. The sequence corresponds to the sequence in which the haplotype arrays are listed. Thus in Table II-1 (p. 00) the Ainu sample from Hokkaido may be explained by an array of haplotypes that includes $Gm^{1,2}$ or one that does not have $Gm^{1,2}$. The arrays are listed under haplotypes with the array including $Gm^{1,2}$ first; the expected phenotype frequencies are listed in the same sequence.

The data for each allotype system (i.e. Gm, Inv, Am) are arranged by race with the races listed alphabetically. Populations within a race that were tested for the same allotypes are listed as a group and are arranged by continent, and by country. Populations within a group and from the same country are listed alphabetically.

The tables are numbered as follows: a Roman numeral is assigned to all tables for a given race within an allotype system. Within a race, all populations tested for a given set of allotypes are assigned to a table with the same Latin numeral added to the Roman numeral. Thus the data for the several populations of Australian Aborigines tested for Gm(1,2,5,6) will be found in Table I-1; the data for those tested for Gm(1,2,3,5,13) will be found in Table I-2, etc.

Table 6 Values of χ^2 corresponding to P = 0.05 and 0.01

Degrees of freedom	P	
	0.05	0.01
1	3.841	6.635
2	5.991	9.210
3	7.851	11.345
4	9.488	13.277
5	11.070	15.086
6	12.592	16.821
7	14.067	18.475
8	15.507	20.090
9	16.919	21.666
10	18.307	23.209

TABLE I-1
TESTED FOR GM 1, 2, 5, 6

PHENOTYPES | HAPLOTYPES

ABORIGINES

OCEANIA

AUSTRALIA

	TOTAL		1	1 2	1 5	1 2 5	1 5	CHI SQ. DF	VALUE		1	1 2	1 5	1 5	REF.
CENTRAL REGION	295	O.	147	148				0		F.	0.706	0.294			92
		E.	147.0	148.0						S.E.	0.021	0.021			
KIMBERLEYS	268	O.	83	103	65	17		1	2.870	F.	0.572	0.259	0.169		188
		E.	87.7	97.6	59.3	23.4				S.E.	0.023	0.020	0.017		
QUEENSLAND															
AURUNKUN	70	O.	39	31				0		F.	0.746	0.254			159
		E.	39.0	31.0						S.E.	0.040	0.040			
EDWARD RIVER	81	O.	56	24	1	0		0		F.	0.833	0.161	0.006		159
		E.	56.1	23.9	0.8	0.2				S.E.	0.031	0.030	0.006		
MITCHELL RIVER	111	O.	81	20	9	1		1	0.000	F.	0.854	0.100	0.046		159
		E.	81.0	20.0	9.0	1.0				S.E.	0.024	0.021	0.014		
NORTH *	103	O.	46	33	18	5	1	2	0.272	F.	0.673	0.206		0.121	29
		E.	46.6	32.9	16.8	5.1	1.5			S.E.	0.034	0.030		0.023	
YARRABAH	88	O.	33	48	5	2		1	0.137	F.	0.616	0.344	0.041		159
		E.	33.4	47.6	4.6	2.5				S.E.	0.041	0.040	0.015		
WESTERN DESERT	289	O.	154	135				0		F.	0.730	0.270			188
		E.	154.0	135.0						S.E.	0.020	0.020			

* NOT TESTED FOR GM(6).

TABLE I-2
TESTED FOR GM 1, 2, 3, 5, 10

ABORIGINES
OCEANIA
AUSTRALIA

PHENOTYPES

	TOTAL		1	1 2	1 5 10	1 2 5 10	DF	CHI SQ. VALUE
KIMBERLEYS	74	O.	24	26	21	3	1	2.346
		E.	26.2	23.4	18.4	6.0		

HAPLOTYPES

		1	1 2	1 5 10	REF.
	F.	0.595	0.224	0.181	128
	S.E.	0.044	0.037	0.033	

TABLE I-3
TESTED FOR GM 1, 2, 3, 5, 6, 13, 14, 21

ABORIGINES
OCEANIA
AUSTRALIA

PHENOTYPES

	TOTAL		21	1 21	1 2 21	1 5 13 14 21	1 2 5 13 14 21	1 5 13 14	DF	CHI SQ. VALUE
BENTINCK ISLAND	33	O.	19	13	1	0	0		0	0
		E.	19.2	12.8	0.8	0.2	0.0			
MORNINGTON ISLAND	89	O.	26	24	31	8	0		2	7.892
		E.	30.1	24.2	22.7	7.8	4.3			
CENTRAL REGION OF N. TERRITORY	84	O.	53	31					0	0
		E.	53.0	31.0						
NORTH REGION OF N. TERRITORY	96	O.	40	40	9	4	3		1	1.017
		E.	38.8	39.1	12.1	5.0	0.9			
S. COAST OF GULF OF CARPENTERIA	128	O.	31	39	29	23	6		2	2.757
		E.	28.7	43.3	30.3	17.7	8.0			

HAPLOTYPES

		21	1 21	1 2 21	1 5 13 14	REF.
	F.	0.763	0.222	0.015		168
	S.E.	0.056	0.055	0.015		
	F.	0.581	0.200	0.219		168
	S.E.	0.038	0.032	0.031		
	F.	0.794	0.206			166
	S.E.	0.033	0.033			
	F.	0.636	0.265	0.099		166
	S.E.	0.037	0.035	0.022		
	F.	0.473	0.277	0.250		168
	S.E.	0.033	0.030	0.027		

17

TABLE I-4
TESTED FOR GM 1, 2, 3, 5, 6, 10, 11, 13, 14, 15, 16, 17, 21, 23, 24

PHENOTYPES

ABORIGINES — OCEANIA — AUSTRALIA

	TOTAL		1 17 21	1 17 21 23	1 2 17 21	1 2 17 21 23	1 5 10 11 13 14 17 21 23	1 5 10 11 13 14 17 21	1 2 5 10 11 13 14 17 21 23	1 5 10 11 13 14 17 21	1 5 10 11 13 14 17 23	DF	CHI SQ. VALUE	REF.
BENTINCK ISLAND	46	O.	0				8		0		38	0		19
		E.	0.3				7.3		0.3		38.3			
MORNINGTON ISLAND	113	O.	45		9		41	3	6	0	9	2	0.920	19
		E.	44.9		10.3		40.4	2.5	4.4	0.0	10.2			
WESTERN DESERT	70	O.	44	19		5	2					1	13.036	19
		E.	44.0	19.0		5.0	2.0							
		E.	40.8	22.3		1.3	5.6							

HAPLOTYPES

ABORIGINES — OCEANIA — AUSTRALIA

	TOTAL		1 17 21	1 2 17 21	1 17 21 23	1 5 10 11 13 14 17 23	1 5 10 11 13 14 17 23	REF.
BENTINCK ISLAND	46	F.	0.087			0.913		19
		S.E.	0.029			0.029		
MORNINGTON ISLAND	113	F.	0.631	0.068		0.018	0.283	19
		S.E.	0.032	0.017		0.010	0.030	
WESTERN DESERT	70	F.	0.793	0.018	0.156	0.033		19
		S.E.	0.036	0.012	0.033	0.016		
		F.	0.763	0.050	0.186	0.035		
		S.E.	0.038	0.019	0.035			

TABLE II-1
TESTED FOR GM 1, 2, 3, 5, 6, 13, 14

PHENOTYPES

AINU

ASIA

JAPAN

	TOTAL	1	1 2	2	1 2 13	1 13	DF	CHI SQ. VALUE	REF.
HOKKAIDO	187	O. 55	30	2	82	18			163
		E. 54.3	30.8	2.1	82.8	17.1	1	0.089	
		E. 55.4	28.3	3.6	83.2	16.5	2	0.987	

HAPLOTYPES

	1	1 2	2	1 13
F.	0.539	0.039	0.105	0.317
S.E.	0.029	0.038	0.036	0.027
F.	0.544		0.139	0.317
S.E.	0.028		0.018	0.027

TABLE II-2
TESTED FOR GM 1, 2, 3, 5, 6, 13, 14, 21

PHENOTYPES

AINU

ASIA

JAPAN

	TOTAL	1 21	1 2 21	2 21	1 3 5 13 14 21	1 3 5 13 14 21	1 2 3 5 13 14 21	1 3 5 13 21 14	1 3 5 13 21 13	1 13 21 13	DF	CHI SQ. VALUE	REF.
HOKKAIDO	159	O. 41	34	2	4	1	3	46	18	10			165
		E. 41.4	34.7	2.0	4.2	1.6	2.3	44.3	16.6	11.9	4	0.895	
		E. 43.3	29.8	5.1	4.2	1.5	2.3	45.3	15.6	11.9	5	3.657	

HAPLOTYPES

	1 21	1 2 21	2 21	1 3 5 13 14 21	1 13	REF.
F.	0.510	0.077	0.113	0.026	0.273	165
S.E.	0.029	0.042	0.039	0.009	0.025	
F.	0.522		0.179	0.026	0.273	
S.E.	0.028		0.022	0.009	0.025	

19

TABLE II-3
TESTED FOR GM 1, 2, 3, 5, 13, 15, 16, 21

PHENOTYPES

AINU
 ASIA
  JAPAN

	TOTAL	1 / 21 21	1 2 / 21 21	1 / 21 21	1 3 5 13 / 13 21	1 2 3 5 13 / 13 21	1 3 5 13 / 13	1 3 5 13 15 16 / 13	1 3 13 15 16 21 / 21	1 2 13 15 16 21 / 21	1 13 15 16 / 21	CHI SQ. DF	VALUE	REF.
HOKKAIDO	407	O. 132	71	1	19	4	2	9	111	32	26			
		E. 128.8	72.6	1.0	20.3	5.1	0.8	9.0	114.8	29.1	25.6	4	1.630	80
HIDAKA		E. 132.8	62.3	7.3	20.6	4.8	0.8	9.0	116.5	27.3	25.6	5	7.883	

HAPLOTYPES

AINU
 ASIA
  JAPAN

	TOTAL	1 / 21 21	1 2 / 21 21	1 2 / 21 21	1 3 5 13 16	1 13 15 16	REF.
HOKKAIDO	407	F. 0.563	0.093	0.050	0.044	0.251	
		S.E. 0.018	0.027	0.025	0.007	0.015	80
HIDAKA		F. 0.571		0.134	0.044	0.251	
		S.E. 0.017		0.012	0.007	0.015	

20

TABLE III-1
TESTED FOR GM 1, 2, 3

PHENOTYPES

	TOTAL	3	1 3	1 2 3	1 2	CHI SQ. DF	VALUE
CAUCASOIDS							
EUROPE							
AUSTRIA							
VIENNA	1602	O. 874	442	55	180	49	
		E. 879.5	439.3	54.8	175.7	52.7	2 0.390
GERMANY							
BERLIN	102	O. 63	19	2	14	4	
		E. 62.0	20.2	1.6	14.9	3.3	2 0.357
POLAND							
LOWER SILESIA	300	O. 182	66	14	30	8	
		E. 176.3	77.2	8.4	30.1	7.9	2 5.455

HAPLOTYPES

		3	1	1 2	REF.
VIENNA	F.	0.741	0.185	0.074	86
	S.E.	0.008	0.007	0.005	
BERLIN	F.	0.779	0.127	0.094	103
	S.E.	0.029	0.024	0.021	
LOWER SILESIA	F.	0.767	0.168	0.066	148
	S.E.	0.017	0.015	0.010	

TABLE III-2
TESTED FOR GM 1, 2, 5

PHENOTYPES / HAPLOTYPES

	TOTAL		5	1 5	5 1	1 2 5	1 2	DF	CHI SQ VALUE		5	1	1 2	1 5	REF.
CAUCASOIDS															
ASIA															
INDIA															
KUMAON REGION															
BRAHAMINS	102	O.	23	55	7	14	3	1	1.421	F.	0.479	0.240	0.086	0.195	17
		E.	23.4	56.0	5.9	11.8	4.9			S.E.	0.043	0.044	0.020	0.056	
DOMS	79	O.	10	40	9	15	5	1	2.333	F.	0.363	0.304	0.132	0.200	17
		E.	10.4	41.7	7.3	11.8	7.7			S.E.	0.052	0.048	0.028	0.064	
RAJPUTS	129	O.	18	67	16	21	7	1	3.351	F.	0.380	0.323	0.113	0.184	17
		E.	18.7	69.5	13.5	16.4	11.0			S.E.	0.041	0.038	0.020	0.050	
TAMILS	132	O.	6	30	41	17	38	2	1.222	F.	0.223	0.543	0.234		66
		E.	6.6	32.0	38.9	13.8	40.7			S.E.	0.026	0.032	0.028		
PAKISTAN															
PESHAWAR	135	O.	41	64	8	20	2	1	4.203	F.	0.558	0.211	0.083	0.149	191
		E.	42.0	65.6	6.0	15.8	5.6			S.E.	0.036	0.038	0.017	0.047	
EUROPE															
CZECHOSLOVAKIA															
OVCIE	507	O.	311	135	10	46	5	2	3.991	F.	0.792	0.157	0.051		149
		E.	318.0	126.2	12.5	40.9	9.4			S.E.	0.013	0.011	0.007		
POLOMA	415	O.	217	166	9	12	11	2	18.409	F.	0.737	0.234	0.028		149
		E.	225.6	143.3	22.8	17.4	5.9			S.E.	0.015	0.015	0.006		
OMITTING GM(2)	415	O.	217	178	20			1	4.784	F.	0.737	0.263			
		E.	225.6	160.7	28.6					S.E.	0.015	0.015			
PRAGUE	192	O.	103	59	7	21	2	2	3.101	F.	0.745	0.195	0.061		122
		E.	106.5	55.7	7.3	17.3	5.2			S.E.	0.022	0.020	0.012		
DENMARK															
DANES	1000	O.	441	280	47	162	70	2	0.152	F.	0.662	0.214	0.124		93
		E.	438.2	283.5	45.9	164.0	68.4			S.E.	0.011	0.009	0.008		

TABLE III-2 CONTINUED
TESTED FOR GM 1,2,5

CAUCASOIDS
EUROPE
FINLAND

PHENOTYPES

POPULATION		TOTAL	5	1/5	5/1	1/2/5	1/2	CHI SQ DF	VALUE
ALAND ISLANDS KOKAR ISLAND	O.	219	89	67	27	29	7	2	9.842
	E.		85.7	79.5	18.4	23.1	12.3		
' OMITTING GM(2)	O.	219	89	96	34			1	0.905
	E.		85.7	102.6	30.7				
HELSINKI	O.	160	67	43	7	26	17	2	1.463
	E.		64.4	44.2	7.6	30.0	13.8		
MAINLAND	O.	333	116	104	25	53	35	2	0.368
	E.		113.6	106.1	24.8	55.6	32.8		
FRANCE									
BEARN	O.	50	18	20	1	7	4	2	2.781
	E.		19.8	15.9	3.2	7.4	3.7		
BRITTANY	O.	100	49	32	2	13	4	2	1.554
	E.		51.1	28.1	3.9	12.7	4.3		
COMMERCY	O.	1236	607	366	46	161	56	2	0.984
	E.		613.1	354.7	51.3	160.1	56.8		
FRENCH	O.	297	168	79	6	43	1	2	10.468
	E.		176.6	70.8	7.1	34.1	8.5		
' OMITTING GM(2)	O.	297	168	122	7			1	7.933
	E.		176.6	104.9	15.6				
LYON	O.	325	165	96	9	44	11	2	1.883
	E.		169.9	88.9	11.6	41.3	13.3		
NORMANDY	O.	1451	693	451	58	187	62	2	2.635
	E.		705.8	431.2	65.9	181.2	67.0		

HAPLOTYPES

POPULATION		5	1	1 2	1 5	REF.
ALAND ISLANDS KOKAR ISLAND	F.	0.626	0.290	0.084		181
	S.E.	0.023	0.022	0.014		
' OMITTING GM(2)	F.	0.626	0.374			
	S.E.	0.023	0.023			
HELSINKI	F.	0.634	0.218	0.148		122
	S.E.	0.027	0.024	0.021		
MAINLAND	F.	0.584	0.273	0.143		181
	S.E.	0.019	0.018	0.014		
BEARN	F.	0.630	0.252	0.118		134
	S.E.	0.048	0.044	0.033		
BRITTANY	F.	0.715	0.196	0.089		134
	S.E.	0.032	0.028	0.021		
COMMERCY	F.	0.704	0.204	0.092		65
	S.E.	0.009	0.008	0.006		
FRENCH	F.	0.771	0.155	0.074		126
	S.E.	0.017	0.015	0.011		
' OMITTING GM(2)	F.	0.771	0.229			
	S.E.	0.017	0.017			
LYON	F.	0.723	0.189	0.088		122
	S.E.	0.018	0.016	0.011		
NORMANDY	F.	0.697	0.213	0.090		127
	S.E.	0.009	0.008	0.005		

TABLE III-2 CONTINUED
TESTED FOR GM 1,2,5

PHENOTYPES

CAUCASOIDS	TOTAL		5	1 5	5 1	1 2 5	1 2	CHI SQ. DF	VALUE	REF.
EUROPE										
FRANCE										
PARIS	705	O.	347	211	30	84	33	2	0.234	88
		E.	346.9	209.3	31.6	86.0	31.3			
ROUSSILLON										
MOUNTAINS	118	O.	50	47	2	15	4	1	0.090	134
		E.	49.8	46.9	2.2	15.5	3.6			
PLAINS	437	O.	208	152	27	37	13	2	0.199	134
		E.	209.4	150.6	27.1	35.6	14.3			
SEINE-MARITIME	746	O.	346	240	28	103	29	2	5.010	120
		E.	359.0	221.9	34.3	95.1	35.7			
TOULOUSE	1023	O.	453	352	50	119	49	2	2.962	134
		E.	463.4	332.2	59.5	118.0	49.8			
TOURS	277	O.	148	80	15	26	8	2	0.925	122
		E.	145.9	84.9	12.3	25.4	8.5			
GERMANY										
FREIBURG	361	O.	201	101	8	42	9	2	1.822	110
		E.	205.7	93.9	10.7	39.7	11.0			
FREIBURG	772	O.	410	230	13	94	25	1	0.665	108
		E.	408.7	229.3	14.4	97.6	22.1			
GERMANS	411	O.	194	120	13	69	15	2	4.318	126
		E.	202.5	110.7	15.1	61.2	21.4			
GERMANS	118	O.	66	37	1	14	0	2	7.028	126
		E.	71.0	30.2	3.2	10.9	2.7	0		
		E.	66.6	37.3	0.5	12.3	1.3			
HESSEN	270	O.	145	68	6	36	15	2	1.545	197
		E.	143.7	66.8	7.8	39.7	12.0			

HAPLOTYPES

		5	1	1 2	1 5
PARIS	F.	0.701	0.212	0.087	
	S.E.	0.012	0.011	0.008	
MOUNTAINS	F.	0.650	0.137	0.085	0.129
	S.E.	0.035	0.040	0.018	0.048
PLAINS	F.	0.692	0.249	0.059	
	S.E.	0.016	0.015	0.008	
SEINE-MARITIME	F.	0.694	0.214	0.092	
	S.E.	0.012	0.011	0.008	
TOULOUSE	F.	0.673	0.241	0.086	
	S.E.	0.010	0.010	0.006	
TOURS	F.	0.726	0.211	0.063	
	S.E.	0.019	0.017	0.010	
FREIBURG	F.	0.755	0.172	0.073	
	S.E.	0.016	0.014	0.010	
FREIBURG	F.	0.728	0.137	0.081	0.055
	S.E.	0.012	0.016	0.007	0.018
GERMANS	F.	0.702	0.192	0.106	
	S.E.	0.016	0.014	0.011	
GERMANS	F.	0.775	0.165	0.059	
	S.E.	0.027	0.024	0.016	
	F.	0.751	0.064	0.059	0.125
	S.E.	0.030	0.040	0.016	0.046
HESSEN	F.	0.730	0.170	0.101	
	S.E.	0.019	0.016	0.013	

TABLE III-2 CONTINUED
TESTED FOR GM 1,2,5

CAUCASOIDS

EUROPE

PHENOTYPES

	TOTAL		5	1 5	5 1	1 2 5	1 2	CHI SQ DF	VALUE
GERMANY									
LEIPZIG	1207	O.	664	275	68	154	46	2	25.812
		E.	639.4	326.3	41.6	151.9	47.8		
LEIPZIG	208	O.	111	64	1	30	2	0	
		E.	111.5	64.3	0.6	28.4	3.1		
MARBURG	238	O.	130	58	5	31	14	2	2.150
		E.	127.9	57.7	6.5	35.4	10.4		
MUNICH	131	O.	73	29	6	19	4	2	2.174
		E.	71.8	32.7	3.7	17.7	5.1		
RHEINLAND-PFALZ	383	O.	178	115	16	63	11	2	6.134
		E.	186.1	108.6	15.9	53.1	19.3		
GREECE									
ATHENS	297	O.	200	78	9	9	1	2	0.553
		E.	199.6	79.5	7.9	8.2	1.7		
GREEKS	218	O.	116	53	7	39	3	2	6.164
		E.	120.4	51.5	5.5	31.7	8.9		
HUNGARY									
BODROGHALOM	71	O.	44	20	1	6	0	2	2.015
		E.	45.8	17.7	1.7	4.8	1.1		
BUDAPEST *	497	O.	301	135	20	34	7	2	1.308
		E.	299.0	140.6	16.5	32.4	8.5		
CIGAND	162	O.	91	47	0	20	4	2	6.131
		E.	95.7	38.6	3.9	19.1	4.8	0	
		E.	90.2	46.6	0.5	22.2	2.5		

HAPLOTYPES

		5	1	1 2	1 5	REF.
LEIPZIG	F.	0.728	0.186	0.086		43
	S.E.	0.009	0.008	0.006		
LEIPZIG	F.	0.732	0.055	0.079	0.134	59
	S.E.	0.024	0.029	0.013	0.034	
MARBURG	F.	0.733	0.165	0.101		22
	S.E.	0.020	0.017	0.014		
MUNICH	F.	0.740	0.169	0.091		122
	S.E.	0.027	0.023	0.018		
RHEINLAND-PFALZ	F.	0.697	0.203	0.099		125
	S.E.	0.017	0.015	0.011		
ATHENS	F.	0.820	0.163	0.017		122
	S.E.	0.016	0.015	0.005		
GREEKS	F.	0.743	0.159	0.098		193
	S.E.	0.021	0.018	0.015		
BODROGHALOM	F.	0.803	0.155	0.042		194
	S.E.	0.033	0.030	0.017		
BUDAPEST	F.	0.776	0.182	0.042		107
	S.E.	0.013	0.012	0.006		
CIGAND	F.	0.769	0.155	0.077		194
	S.E.	0.023	0.020	0.015		
	F.	0.746	0.057	0.079	0.118	
	S.E.	0.026	0.033	0.015	0.038	

* EXCLUDING THREE GM(-1,-2,-5) SAMPLES.

TABLE III-2 CONTINUED
TESTED FOR GM 1,2,5

CAUCASOIDS

EUROPE

PHENOTYPES

HUNGARY	TOTAL	O./E.	5	1 5	5 1	1 2 5	1 2	DF	CHI SQ. VALUE
DAMOC	72	O.	51	17	0	4	0	1	2.099
		E.	52.5	14.5	1.0	3.4	0.5		
KARCSA	129	O.	92	31	3	3	0	1	0.048
		E.	92.1	31.3	2.7	2.5	0.4		
KENEZLO	56	O.	26	14	0	15	1	1	4.841
		E.	29.3	10.6	1.0	11.8	3.3		
KISROZVAGY	49	O.	23	21	1	3	1	2	2.327
		E.	25.0	17.1	2.9	2.9	1.1		
NAGYROZVAGY	116	O.	70	37	1	7	1	2	2.986
		E.	73.0	31.7	3.4	6.4	1.5		
PACIN	136	O.	69	34	1	29	3	2	5.496
		E.	74.3	28.2	2.7	24.3	6.6		
REVLEANYVAR	81	O.	58	20	1	2	0	1	0.487
		E.	58.8	18.7	1.5	1.7	0.3		
RICSE	75	O.	41	24	3	6	1	2	0.399
		E.	41.8	23.1	3.2	5.3	1.6		
SEMJEN	60	O.	42	17	0	1	0	0	
		E.	43.4	14.5	1.2	0.8	0.1		
TISZAKARAD	76	O.	52	17	1	4	2	1	0.415
		E.	51.4	17.1	1.4	5.1	1.0		
ZEMPLENAGARD	66	O.	37	21	0	8	0	2	5.232
		E.	40.2	16.4	1.7	6.2	1.5		

HAPLOTYPES

HUNGARY		5	1	1 2	1 5	REF.
DAMOC	F.	0.854	0.118	0.028		194
	S.E.	0.029	0.027	0.014		
KARCSA	F.	0.845	0.143	0.012		194
	S.E.	0.023	0.022	0.007		
KENEZLO	F.	0.723	0.131	0.146		194
	S.E.	0.042	0.033	0.034		
KISROZVAGY	F.	0.714	0.244	0.042		194
	S.E.	0.046	0.043	0.020		
NAGYROZVAGY	F.	0.793	0.172	0.035		194
	S.E.	0.027	0.025	0.012		
PACIN	F.	0.739	0.140	0.121		194
	S.E.	0.027	0.022	0.020		
REVLEANYVAR	F.	0.852	0.136	0.012		194
	S.E.	0.028	0.027	0.009		
RICSE	F.	0.747	0.206	0.047		194
	S.E.	0.036	0.033	0.018		
SEMJEN	F.	0.850	0.142	0.008		194
	S.E.	0.033	0.032	0.008		
TISZAKARAD	F.	0.822	0.136	0.041		194
	S.E.	0.031	0.028	0.016		
ZEMPLENAGARD	F.	0.780	0.159	0.061		194
	S.E.	0.036	0.032	0.021		

TABLE III-2 CONTINUED
TESTED FOR GM 1,2,5

PHENOTYPES / HAPLOTYPES

CAUCASOIDS
EUROPE

	TOTAL		5	1 5	1 2 5	1	1 2	CHI SQ. DF	VALUE		5	1	1 2	1 5	REF.
ICELAND															
DALASYSLA	190	O.	84	47	42	8	9	2	2.986	F.	0.676	0.183	0.141		95
		E.	86.9	47.0	36.2	6.4	13.6			S.E.	0.024	0.020	0.018		
IRELAND															
IRISH	294	O.	119	76	62	19	18	2	5.176	F.	0.639	0.217	0.144		96
		E.	120.2	81.5	54.0	13.8	24.4			S.E.	0.020	0.017	0.015		
ITALY															
FERRARA	87	O.	55	23	2	3	4	2	7.627	F.	0.776	0.188	0.037		186
		E.	52.4	25.3	4.9	3.1	1.3			S.E.	0.032	0.030	0.014		
′ OMITTING GM(2)	87	O.	55	25		7		1	2.628	F.	0.776	0.224			
		E.	52.4	30.3		4.4				S.E.	0.032	0.032			
LAZIO	180	O.	92	65	14	6	3	2	2.376	F.	0.731	0.221	0.048		24
		E.	96.1	58.2	12.6	8.8	4.2			S.E.	0.023	0.022	0.011		
SICILIANS *	263	O.	140	96	6	18	3	2	0.279	F.	0.726	0.256	0.017		76
		E.	138.7	98.0	6.6	17.3	2.4			S.E.	0.019	0.019	0.006		
NETHERLANDS															
DUTCH	348	O.	159	99	45	14	31	2	5.252	F.	0.664	0.217	0.119		122
		E.	153.3	100.5	54.9	16.5	22.9			S.E.	0.018	0.016	0.013		
NORWAY															
NORWEGIANS	199	O.	78	60	36	7	18	2	1.205	F.	0.633	0.220	0.147		12
		E.	79.8	55.4	37.0	9.6	17.2			S.E.	0.024	0.021	0.018		
NORWEGIANS	680	O.	256	191	141	44	48	2	6.837	F.	0.621	0.232	0.147		47
		E.	261.9	195.7	124.5	36.6	61.3			S.E.	0.013	0.012	0.010		
′ OMITTING GM(2)	680	O.	256	332		92		1	0.920	F.	0.621	0.379			
		E.	261.9	320.2		97.9				S.E.	0.013	0.013			

* EXCLUDING ONE GM(2,5) SAMPLE.

27

TABLE III-2 CONTINUED
TESTED FOR GM 1,2,5

PHENOTYPES

	TOTAL		5	1 5	1	1 2 5	1 2	DF	CHI SQ. VALUE
CAUCASOIDS									
EUROPE									
POLAND									
KRACOW REGION	600	O.	384	140	10	59	7	2	2.561
		E.	389.6	133.6	11.5	54.1	11.2		
YUGOSLAVIA									
LJUBLJANA	157	O.	98	33	3	21	2	2	1.314
		E.	99.5	32.3	2.6	18.7	3.9		
MIDDLE EAST									
IRAN									
CENTRAL AND SOUTH	231	O.	117	72	8	31	3	2	5.431
		E.	122.9	66.0	8.9	25.2	8.0		
EAST	173	O.	88	55	3	23	4	1	0.147
		E.	88.3	55.2	2.7	22.2	4.6		
IRANIANS	298	O.	129	117	29	17	6	2	0.612
		E.	128.9	118.8	27.4	15.4	7.5		
NORTH	169	O.	75	59	12	19	4	2	1.932
		E.	76.9	58.4	11.1	15.8	6.8		
NORTHWEST	233	O.	118	70	11	27	7	2	0.536
		E.	119.0	70.0	10.3	25.1	8.7		
TEHERAN	374	O.	172	144	13	36	9	1	0.133
		E.	172.3	144.3	12.5	35.0	9.9		
TEHERAN - BORN BEFORE 1936	92	O.	49	35	2	5	1	2	2.421
		E.	51.8	29.9	4.3	4.6	1.4		
TEHERAN - BORN 1936 AND AFTER	187	O.	80	81	5	18	3	1	0.356
		E.	80.3	81.3	4.5	16.9	3.9		

HAPLOTYPES

		5	1	1 2	1 5	REF.
KRACOW REGION	F.	0.806	0.138	0.056		151
	S.E.	0.011	0.010	0.007		
LJUBLJANA	F.	0.796	0.129	0.075		122
	S.E.	0.023	0.019	0.015		
CENTRAL AND SOUTH	F.	0.729	0.196	0.075		4
	S.E.	0.021	0.019	0.012		
EAST	F.	0.714	0.125	0.081	0.080	4
	S.E.	0.026	0.033	0.015	0.038	
IRANIANS	F.	0.658	0.303	0.039		119
	S.E.	0.019	0.019	0.008		
NORTH	F.	0.675	0.256	0.069		4
	S.E.	0.025	0.024	0.014		
NORTHWEST	F.	0.715	0.210	0.075		4
	S.E.	0.021	0.019	0.012		
TEHERAN	F.	0.679	0.183	0.062	0.076	4
	S.E.	0.019	0.023	0.009	0.026	
TEHERAN - BORN BEFORE 1936	F.	0.750	0.217	0.033		3
	S.E.	0.032	0.030	0.013		
TEHERAN - BORN 1936 AND AFTER	F.	0.655	0.155	0.057	0.132	3
	S.E.	0.028	0.033	0.012	0.039	

TABLE III-2 CONTINUED
TESTED FOR GM 1,2,5

PHENOTYPES

	TOTAL		5	1 5	1	1 2 5	1 2	CHI SQ. DF	VALUE
CAUCASOIDS									
MIDDLE EAST									
IRAN									
WEST	300	O.	142	99	12	35	17	2	1.111
		E.	145.6	92.8	14.8	34.0	12.8		
N. AMERICA									
CUBA									
SANTIAGO DE CUBA *	181	O.	28	124	11	13	5	1	0.000
		E.	28.0	124.0	11.0	13.0	5.0		
U.S.A.									
OAKLAND, CA.	478	O.	183	168	27	75	25	2	4.949
		E.	194.0	154.5	30.8	66.5	32.7		
OCEANIA									
AUSTRALIA									
MIXED, MAINLY BRITISH	300	O.	130	91	20	37	27	2	1.418
		E.	175.5	96.5	18.5	40.6	18.9		

HAPLOTYPES

		5	1	1 2	1 5	REF.
WEST	F.	0.697	0.222	0.081		4
	S.E.	0.019	0.017	0.011		
SANTIAGO DE CUBA *	F.	0.393	0.246	0.051	0.309	52
	S.E.	0.034	0.034	0.012	0.045	
OAKLAND, CA.	F.	0.637	0.254	0.109		106
	S.E.	0.016	0.014	0.010		
MIXED, MAINLY BRITISH	F.	0.647	0.249	0.105		189
	S.E.	0.020	0.018	0.013		

* EXCLUDING ONE GM(2,5) SAMPLE.

29

TABLE III-3
TESTED FOR GM 1, 2, 11

PHENOTYPES

CAUCASOIDS
EUROPE

SCOTLAND	TOTAL		1 1	1 1	1	1 2 / 1 1	1	1 2	DF	CHI SQ VALUE
BLACK ISLE	136	O.	61	41	9	16	9		2	0.656
		E.	58.9	43.8	8.1	17.4	7.8			
EAST COAST SUTHERLAND	208	O.	103	53	5	33	14		2	0.891
		E.	102.5	51.5	6.5	35.5	12.0			
EASTER ROSS	368	O.	164	102	11	61	30		2	1.956
		E.	163.8	97.7	14.6	65.7	26.2			
GREAT GLEN AND E. TO RIV. SPEY	343	O.	149	108	19	51	16		2	1.265
		E.	152.2	106.0	18.5	46.6	19.8			
W. SIDE, GREAT GLEN, LOCHABER	301	O.	140	81	12	53	15		2	0.919
		E.	142.4	80.1	11.3	49.2	18.1			
INLAND ROSS AND CROMARTY	352	O.	156	112	11	54	19		2	3.009
		E.	162.3	101.2	15.8	52.2	20.5			
INVERNESS TOWN	633	O.	289	175	23	106	40		2	0.295
		E.	291.4	170.7	25.0	105.5	40.4			
MORAY COAST	592	O.	263	172	18	101	38		2	2.484
		E.	269.6	159.9	23.7	99.9	38.9			
NORTH CAITHNESS	211	O.	75	68	16	39	13		2	2.609
		E.	78.3	67.2	14.4	33.2	17.8			
ORKNEY ISLANDS	154	O.	61	56	6	25	6		2	4.488
		E.	66.9	48.1	8.6	21.1	9.3			

HAPLOTYPES

		1 1	1	1 2	REF.
BLACK ISLE	F.	0.658	0.245	0.097	61
	S.E.	0.029	0.026	0.018	
EAST COAST SUTHERLAND	F.	0.702	0.176	0.122	61
	S.E.	0.022	0.019	0.016	
EASTER ROSS	F.	0.667	0.199	0.134	61
	S.E.	0.017	0.015	0.013	
GREAT GLEN AND E. TO RIV. SPEY	F.	0.666	0.232	0.102	61
	S.E.	0.018	0.016	0.012	
W. SIDE, GREAT GLEN, LOCHABER	F.	0.688	0.193	0.119	61
	S.E.	0.019	0.016	0.014	
INLAND ROSS AND CROMARTY	F.	0.679	0.212	0.109	61
	S.E.	0.018	0.016	0.012	
INVERNESS TOWN	F.	0.679	0.199	0.123	61
	S.E.	0.013	0.011	0.009	
MORAY COAST	F.	0.675	0.200	0.125	61
	S.E.	0.014	0.012	0.010	
NORTH CAITHNESS	F.	0.609	0.262	0.129	61
	S.E.	0.024	0.022	0.017	
ORKNEY ISLANDS	F.	0.659	0.237	0.104	61
	S.E.	0.027	0.025	0.018	

TABLE III-3 CONTINUED
TESTED FOR GM 1,2,11

PHENOTYPES

CAUCASOIDS

EUROPE

SCOTLAND

	TOTAL		1 1	1 1	1	1 2 1 1	1 2	DF	CHI SQ. VALUE
SHETLAND ISLANDS	146	O.	62	39	11	29	5	2	6.279
		E.	63.1	42.7	7.2	23.1	9.9		
OMITTING GM(2)	146	O.	62	68	16			1	0.170
		E.	63.1	65.8	17.1				
STRATHGLASS AND ABRIACHAN	106	O.	46	33	2	13	12	2	5.728
		E.	44.9	30.1	5.0	18.1	7.9		

HAPLOTYPES

		1 1	1	1 2	REF.
SHETLAND ISLANDS	F.	0.658	0.222	0.120	61
	S.E.	0.028	0.025	0.020	
OMITTING GM(2)	F.	0.658	0.342		
	S.E.	0.028	0.028		
STRATHGLASS AND ABRIACHAN	F.	0.651	0.218	0.131	61
	S.E.	0.033	0.029	0.024	

TABLE III-4
TESTED FOR GM 1,3,5

PHENOTYPES

CAUCASOIDS

EUROPE

SWEDEN

	TOTAL		3 5	1 3 5	1	1 5	1 3	DF	CHI SQ. VALUE
SWEDES	560	O.	235	248	75	1	1	0	
		E.	230.1	257.7	70.3	0.9	0.9		
*	558	O.	235	248	75			1	0.553
		E.	231.0	256.1	71.0				

N. AMERICA

U.S.A.

	TOTAL		3 5	1 3 5	1	1 5	1 3	DF	CHI SQ. VALUE
BOSTON, MA.	313	O.	135	135	43			1	0.975
		E.	131.0	143.0	39.0				

HAPLOTYPES

		3 5	1	1 5	1 3	REF.
SWEDES	F.	0.641	0.354	0.002	0.002	74
	S.E.	0.014	0.015	0.002	0.002	
*	F.	0.643	0.357			
	S.E.	0.014	0.014			
BOSTON, MA.	F.	0.647	0.353			67
	S.E.	0.019	0.019			

* EXCLUDING ONE GM(1,5) AND ONE GM(1,3) SAMPLES.

TABLE III-5
TESTED FOR GM 1, 2, 3, 5

PHENOTYPES

		Total	3 5	1 3 5	1	1 2 3 5	1 2	1 5	1 2 5	1 3	1 2 3	DF	CHI SQ. VALUE	REF.
CAUCASOIDS														
ASIA														
INDIA														
MADRAS	O.	134	22	57	22	15	16	1	1			2	1.336	45
	E.		25.1	51.0	24.3	14.8	16.7	1.7	0.5					
EUROPE														
CZECHOSLOVAKIA														
BRNO	O.	875	516	211	27	103	18	1	0			1	3.397	56
	E.		517.0	216.4	22.0	95.5	24.1	0.6	0.3					
GERMANY														
BAYERISCHEN WALD	O.	2000	979	581	59	277	91	4	2	4	3	4	2.873	201
	E.		991.1	557.8	68.8	276.0	91.9	4.4	2.3	5.1	2.7			
HESSEN *	O.	1997	977	550	72	282	101	7	5	3	0	4	2.264	199
	E.		971.6	557.0	70.2	285.8	97.8	7.6	4.0	1.9	1.0			
LEIPZIG	O.	2087	1193	508	63	250	64	3	6			3	7.952	44
	E.		1184.1	525.1	52.8	250.7	66.2	5.5	2.7					
L.INDAU	O.	1300	633	372	49	174	63	2	2	3	2	4	0.704	201
	E.		631.4	372.5	48.8	176.8	61.5	2.7	1.3	3.3	1.6			
SCHLESWIG-HOLSTEIN	O.	2000	964	537	69	303	114	3	4	2	4	4	3.960	201
	E.		957.7	540.1	68.0	312.6	108.8	4.3	2.6	3.7	2.2			
SUDLICHEN EIFEL #	O.	2249	1053	653	108	296	121	3	2	8	5	4	2.890	201
	E.		1037.4	676.5	98.7	303.7	115.9	3.2	1.5	8.2	3.8			
UNTERFRANKEN, OBERFRANKEN	O.	3000	1588	796	103	376	121	9	2	4	1	4	2.964	201
	E.		1575.3	817.8	95.9	379.5	116.5	7.0	3.3	3.1	1.5			
WURZBURG	O.	2000	1027	561	62	260	83	4	1	2	0	3	1.177	200
	E.		1033.2	549.7	68.1	259.0	82.7	3.6	1.7	1.4	0.7			

* EXCLUDING THREE GM(2,3,5) SAMPLES.

EXCLUDING ONE GM(2,3,5) SAMPLE.

32

	TOTAL		3 5	1	1 2	1 5	1 3	REF.
CAUCASOIDS								
ASIA								
INDIA								
MADRAS	134	F.	0.433	0.425	0.127	0.015		45
		S.E.	0.030	0.031	0.021	0.010		
EUROPE								
CZECHOSLOVAKIA								
BRNO	875	F.	0.768	0.159	0.071	0.002		56
		S.E.	0.010	0.009	0.006	0.002		
GERMANY								
BAYERISCHEN WALD	2000	F.	0.704	0.185	0.098	0.006	0.007	201
		S.E.	0.007	0.007	0.005	0.002	0.002	
HESSEN	1997	F.	0.698	0.188	0.103	0.010	0.003	199
		S.E.	0.007	0.007	0.005	0.003	0.001	
LEIPZIG	2087	F.	0.753	0.159	0.080	0.008		44
		S.E.	0.007	0.006	0.004	0.003		
LINDAU	1300	F.	0.697	0.194	0.098	0.005	0.006	201
		S.E.	0.009	0.009	0.006	0.003	0.003	
SCHLESWIG-HOLSTEIN	2000	F.	0.692	0.184	0.113	0.006	0.005	201
		S.E.	0.007	0.007	0.005	0.002	0.002	
SUDLICHEN EIFEL	2249	F.	0.679	0.210	0.099	0.003	0.009	201
		S.E.	0.007	0.007	0.005	0.002	0.002	
UNTERFRANKEN, OBERFRANKEN	3000	F.	0.725	0.179	0.087	0.006	0.003	201
		S.E.	0.006	0.005	0.004	0.002	0.001	
WURZBURG	2000	F.	0.719	0.184	0.090	0.005	0.002	200
		S.E.	0.007	0.007	0.005	0.002	0.001	

TABLE III-5 CONTINUED
TESTED FOR GM 1, 2, 3, 5

PHENOTYPES

CAUCASOIDS
EUROPE
GREECE

		TOTAL		3 5	1 3 5	3 1	1 2 3 5	1 2	1 5	1 2 5	DF	CHI SQ. VALUE	REF.
ACHAIA, N. W. PELOPONNESUS *	149	O.	95	43	4	3	2	2	0			
		E.	93.4	45.1	3.9	4.0	0.9	1.6	0.2	2	1.462	2
GREEKS *	252	O.	173	66	6	5	0	2	0			
		E.	172.5	67.8	5.0	4.1	0.7	1.7	0.1	1	0.533	2

HAPLOTYPES

		3 5	3 1	1 2	1 5
	F.	0.792	0.161	0.017	0.030
	S. E.	0.024	0.028	0.008	0.021
	F.	0.827	0.141	0.010	0.022
	S. E.	0.017	0.021	0.004	0.015

* EXCLUDING TWO GM(1,3) SAMPLES.

TABLE III-6
TESTED FOR GM 1, 2, 5, 6

PHENOTYPES — HAPLOTYPES

			5	1 5	1	1 2 5	1 2	1 5 6	1 2 5 6	CHI SQ. DF	VALUE	5	1	1 2	1 5	1 5 6	REF.
CAUCASOIDS																	
ASIA																	
CEYLON	TOTAL																
SINHALESE COLOMBO	159	O.	11	47	43	11	47			2	3.042	F. 0.252	0.542	0.206			188
		E.	10.1	43.4	46.8	16.5	42.3					S.E. 0.024	0.029	0.024			
TAMILS NO. CENT. PROV.	108	O.	5	32	39	9	23			2	0.326	F. 0.236	0.603	0.161			188
		E.	6.0	30.8	39.3	8.2	23.7					S.E. 0.029	0.034	0.026			
VEDDAHS	52	O.	19	23	6	1	3			2	2.255	F. 0.596	0.364	0.040			188
		E.	18.5	22.6	6.9	2.5	1.6					S.E. 0.048	0.047	0.019			
WANNI CASTE NO. CENT. PROV.	98	O.	11	49	10	9	19			2	13.146	F. 0.408	0.434	0.158			188
		E.	16.3	34.7	18.5	12.6	15.9			1	5.125	S.E. 0.035	0.036	0.027			
		E.	10.2	45.6	13.3	14.8	14.1					F. 0.323	0.368	0.160	0.148		
												S.E. 0.047	0.042	0.027	0.056		
INDIA																	
IRULAS NILGIRI HILLS	74	O.	22	22	14	12	4			2	5.865	F. 0.527	0.361	0.112			188
		E.	20.6	28.2	9.7	8.7	6.9					S.E. 0.041	0.040	0.027			
KURUMBAS NILGIRI HILLS	52	O.	14	24	7	4	3			2	0.396	F. 0.538	0.392	0.070			188
		E.	15.1	21.9	8.0	3.9	3.1					S.E. 0.049	0.048	0.025			
TODAS NILGIRI HILLS	99	O.	57	30	4	5	3			2	0.955	F. 0.753	0.206	0.042			188
		E.	56.1	30.6	4.2	6.2	1.9					S.E. 0.031	0.029	0.014			
ORAONS BIHAR	124	O.	11	105	4	3	1			0		F. 0.298	0.183	0.016	0.503		188
		E.	11.0	104.9	4.1	3.2	0.8					S.E. 0.043	0.043	0.008	0.059		
MALAYSIA																	
INDIANS KUALA LUMPUR	128	O.	6	30	39	17	36			2	1.302	F. 0.230	0.538	0.232			152
		E.	6.8	31.7	37.0	13.7	38.8					S.E. 0.026	0.033	0.028			

TABLE III-6 CONTINUED
TESTED FOR GM 1, 2, 5, 6

PHENOTYPES

	TOTAL		5	1 5	5 1	1 2 5	1 2	1 5 6	1 2 5 6	DF	CHI SQ. VALUE
CAUCASOIDS											
ASIA											
PAKISTAN											
PATHANS PESHAWAR	109	O.	38	40	12	11	8			2	0.169
		E.	37.0	41.4	11.6	11.6	7.4				
PUNJABI LAHORE	203	O.	61	87	24	15	16			2	1.749
		E.	61.8	82.4	27.5	18.0	13.3				
EUROPE											
FRANCE											
BASQUES	94	O.	43	32	5	11	3			2	0.478
		E.	44.3	30.6	5.3	9.9	4.0				
GREECE											
ATHENS	504	O.	326	138	19	16	5			2	1.109
		E.	322.2	144.5	16.2	17.0	4.0				
GHAVRIA ARTA PREFECTURE	340	O.	248	79	4			9		1	0.683
		E.	249.7	75.6	5.7			9.0			
KALOVATOS ARTA PREFECTURE *	313	O.	140	140	8	18	0	7	0	1	4.178
		E.	141.0	141.0	6.5	14.7	2.8	6.8	0.2		
POLAND											
POZNAN	305	O.	193	77	6	24	5			2	0.292
		E.	194.4	74.5	7.1	23.7	5.3				
YUGOSLAVIA											
METKOVIK, STON AND DUBROVNIK	121	O.	81	28	3	8	1			2	0.302
		E.	81.0	28.5	2.5	7.5	1.5				
RIJEKA	134	O.	84	36	2	11	1			2	1.533
		E.	86.2	32.8	3.1	9.7	2.1				

HAPLOTYPES

		5	1	1 2	1 5	1 5 6	REF.
PATHANS PESHAWAR	F.	0.583	0.326	0.092			188
	S.E.	0.033	0.032	0.020			
PUNJABI LAHORE	F.	0.552	0.368	0.080			188
	S.E.	0.025	0.024	0.014			
BASQUES	F.	0.686	0.237	0.077			102
	S.E.	0.034	0.031	0.020			
ATHENS	F.	0.800	0.179	0.021			102
	S.E.	0.013	0.012	0.005			
GHAVRIA ARTA PREFECTURE	F.	0.857	0.130			0.013	32
	S.E.	0.014	0.013			0.004	
KALOVATOS ARTA PREFECTURE *	F.	0.671	0.144	0.029	0.145	0.011	32
	S.E.	0.021	0.027	0.007	0.031	0.004	
POZNAN	F.	0.798	0.153	0.049			102
	S.E.	0.016	0.015	0.009			
METKOVIK, STON AND DUBROVNIK	F.	0.818	0.144	0.038			30
	S.E.	0.025	0.023	0.012			
RIJEKA	F.	0.802	0.153	0.045			30
	S.E.	0.024	0.022	0.013			

* EXCLUDING ONE GM(2,5) SAMPLE.

TABLE III-6 CONTINUED
TESTED FOR GM 1,2,5,6

PHENOTYPES

CAUCASOIDS		TOTAL		5	1 5	5 1	1 2 5	1 2	1 5 6	1 2 5 6	CHI SQ. DF	CHI SQ. VALUE
EUROPE												
YUGOSLAVIA												
SPLIT, BIOGRAD AND ZADAR	197	O.	141	42	3	11	0			2	1.834
		E.	142.4	40.8	2.9	9.4	1.5				
MIDDLE EAST												
IRAN												
IRANIANS	296	O.	139	106	22	18	11			2	0.907
		E.	136.5	108.7	21.6	20.3	8.9				
N. AMERICA												
U.S.A.												
CLAXTON, GA.	295	O.	134	88	21	38	12	2	0	2	2.282
		E.	132.5	94.3	16.8	34.8	14.6	1.8	0.2		
CLEVELAND, OH.	303	O.	149	87	14	42	11			2	0.973
		E.	150.4	87.4	12.7	38.8	13.7				
OCEANIA												
AUSTRALIA												
WESTERN REGION	300	O.	130	91	20	37	22			2	1.418
		E.	125.5	96.5	18.5	40.6	18.9				

HAPLOTYPES

		5	1	1 2	1 5	1 5 6	REF.
SPLIT, BIOGRAD AND ZADAR	F.	0.850	0.122	0.028			30
	S.E.	0.018	0.017	0.008			
IRANIANS	F.	0.679	0.270	0.051			101
	S.E.	0.019	0.018	0.009			
CLAXTON, GA.	F.	0.670	0.238	0.088	0.003	0.003	10
	S.E.	0.019	0.018	0.012	0.002	0.002	
CLEVELAND, OH.	F.	0.705	0.205	0.091			153
	S.E.	0.019	0.017	0.012			
WESTERN REGION	F.	0.647	0.249	0.105			188
	S.E.	0.020	0.018	0.013			

TABLE III-7
TESTED FOR GM 1, 2, 3, 5, 10

PHENOTYPES

CAUCASOIDS

EUROPE

FRANCE

	TOTAL		3;5;10	1;3;5;10	1	1;2;3;5;10	1;2	1;5;10	1;2;5;10	1;3	1;2;3	CHI SQ. DF	VALUE	REF.
NORMANDY	129	O.	56	46	4	19	1	1	0	2	0	2	6.463	128
		E.	60.6	42.0	4.2	13.8	4.4	1.0	0.4	1.9	0.7			
NORMANDY *	615	O.	326	166	10	89	18	0	2	4	0	3	4.869	129
		E.	334.3	154.9	12.9	83.6	21.7	1.6	1.0	3.2	1.9			
PARIS	80	O.	34	33	1	5	6	1	0			2	7.227	128
		E.	35.1	27.9	4.2	7.8	3.2	1.2	0.4					
HUNGARY														
BUDAPEST	58	O.	36	14	4	4	0					1	1.250	130
		E.	34.9	17.1	2.1	3.1	0.8							
HEVES	95	O.	62	28	2	3	0					1	0.341	130
		E.	63.2	26.1	2.7	2.4	0.5							
IRAD	112	O.	79	25	3	4	1					1	0.419	130
		E.	78.1	26.7	2.3	4.2	0.8							
ITALY														
BARI #	144	O.	74	58	2	8	0			1	1	2	5.966	128
		E.	79.5	48.3	3.5	6.7	1.5			3.9	0.6			

* EXCLUDING EIGHT GM(5,10) SAMPLES.

EXCLUDING ONE GM(1,2,3,5) SAMPLE.

HAPLOTYPES

	TOTAL		35/10	1	12	15/10	13	REF.
CAUCASOIDS								
EUROPE								
FRANCE								
NORMANDY	129	F.	0.685	0.180	0.078	0.020	0.037	128
		S.E.	0.029	0.033	0.017	0.016	0.021	
NORMANDY	615	F.	0.737	0.145	0.092	0.008	0.017	129
		S.E.	0.013	0.013	0.008	0.005	0.007	
PARIS	80	F.	0.663	0.233	0.074	0.030		128
		S.E.	0.037	0.039	0.021	0.023		
HUNGARY								
BUDAPEST	58	F.	0.776	0.190	0.034			130
		S.E.	0.039	0.036	0.017			
HEVES	95	F.	0.816	0.168	0.016			130
		S.E.	0.028	0.027	0.009			
IRAD	112	F.	0.835	0.143	0.023			130
		S.E.	0.025	0.023	0.010			
ITALY								
BARI	144	F.	0.743	0.155	0.031		0.070	128
		S.E.	0.026	0.033	0.010		0.029	

TABLE III-8
TESTED FOR GM 1, 2, 3, 5, 21

PHENOTYPES

CAUCASOIDS	TOTAL	3 5 21	1 3 5 21	1 3 21	1 2 3 5 21	3 5	1 3 5	CHI SQ. DF	VALUE
EUROPE									
NORWAY									
NORWEGIANS — O.	612	231	178	34	105	56	8	2	0.256
NORWEGIANS — E.		228.7	179.7	34.1	108.2	53.4	7.9		

HAPLOTYPES

	3 5	3 21	1 21	1 2 21	1 3 5	REF.
F.	0.611	0.236	0.142	0.010	0.010	36
S.E.	0.014	0.012	0.010	0.004		

TABLE III-9
TESTED FOR GM 1, 2, 3, 5, 10, 11

PHENOTYPES

CAUCASOIDS	TOTAL	3 5 10 11	1 3 5 10 11	1 3 10 11	1 2 3 5 10 11	1 10 11	CHI SQ. DF	VALUE
EUROPE								
ICELAND								
ICELANDERS * — O.	395	123	120	17	85	50	2	2.981
ICELANDERS * — E.		128.7	108.4	22.8	85.1	49.9		
UNITED KINGDOM								
BRITISH — O.	1000	417	304	54	166	59	2	2.415
BRITISH — E.		425.1	299.2	52.6	154.6	68.5		

HAPLOTYPES

		3 5	10 11 1	1 2	REF.
ICELANDERS	F.	0.571	0.240	0.189	7
	S.E.	0.018	0.016	0.015	
BRITISH	F.	0.652	0.229	0.119	13
	S.E.	0.011	0.010	0.007	

* EXCLUDING ONE GM (1, 5, 10, 11) SAMPLE.

TABLE III-10
TESTED FOR GM 1, 2, 3, 5, 10, 13, 21

PHENOTYPES

		3 5 10 13	1 3 5 10 13 21	1 2 3 5 10 13 21	1 3 5 10 13 21	1 2 21	1 3 5 10 13	CHI SQ. DF VALUE	REF.
CAUCASOIDS									
EUROPE									
PORTUGAL	TOTAL								
PORTUGESE	419 O.	188	136	53	16	9	17	2 5.725	97
	E.	196.3	125.5	45.3	18.4	15.7	17.8		

HAPLOTYPES

		3 5 10 13	1 10 21	1 2 21	1 3 5 10 13
	F.	0.685	0.210	0.076	0.030
	S.E.	0.017	0.014	0.009	0.007

TABLE III-11
TESTED FOR GM 1, 2, 3, 5, 6, 13, 14

PHENOTYPES

		3 5 13 14	1 3 5 13 14	1	1 2 3 5 13 14	1 2 13 14	1 13 14	1 2 13	1 5 13 14	1 2 5 13 14	CHI SQ. DF VALUE	REF.
CAUCASOIDS												
AFRICA												
SOUTH AFRICA	TOTAL											
ASIATIC IND. DURBAN	398 O.	50	137	57	55	63	26	7	2	1	3 1.780	64
	E.	53.6	134.4	58.4	50.5	64.6	23.8	9.8	2.2	0.8		

HAPLOTYPES

		3 5 13 14	1	1 2 13 14	1 5 13 14	1 13 14	REF.
CAUCASOIDS							
AFRICA							
SOUTH AFRICA	TOTAL						
ASIATIC IND. DURBAN	398 F.	0.367	0.383	0.173	0.071	0.006	64
	S.E.	0.017	0.019	0.014	0.012	0.003	

41

TABLE III-12
TESTED FOR GM 1, 2, 3, 5, 10, 11, 21

PHENOTYPES

CAUCASOIDS
  EUROPE
    YUGOSLAVIA

	TOTAL	3;5;10;11	1;3;5;10;11;21	1;2;3;5;10;11;21	1;3;5;10;11;21	1;2;21	1;3;5;10;11;21	1;5;10;11;21	1;2;5;10;11;21	1;5;10;11	CHI SQ. DF	CHI SQ. VALUE	REF.
KOCEVICI * O.	188	75	66	19	18	6	3	1	0	0	3	1.815	132
E.		74.7	69.6	16.2	15.5	8.0	2.5	1.2	0.3	0.0			

HAPLOTYPES

CAUCASOIDS
  EUROPE
    YUGOSLAVIA

	TOTAL	3;5;10;11	1;5;10;11	1;2;21	1;3;5;10;11;21	REF.
KOCEVICI F.	188	0.630	0.294	0.065	0.011	132
S.E.		0.025	0.024	0.013	0.005	

* EXCLUDING ONE GM(1,2,3,5,10,11) SAMPLE.

TABLE III-13
TESTED FOR GM 1, 2, 3, 5, 6, 13, 14, 21

PHENOTYPES

CAUCASOIDS ASIA INDIA	TOTAL	O / E	3 5 13 14	1 3 5 13 14 21	21 21	1 2 5 13 14 21	1 3 5 13 14	1 3 13 21	1 13 21	1 2 13 21	1 13	DF	CHI SQ VALUE	REF
IRANIS *	106	O	42	40	7	10	0	3	4	0	0	3	6.955	173
		E	44.3	37.5	7.9	6.5	3.0	4.5	1.9	0.3	0.1			
EUROPE FINLAND														
ALANDERS ALAND ISLANDS #	117	O	41	34	16	18	4	2	0	2	0	3	7.752	174
		E	39.5	40.3	10.3	14.3	8.6	2.3	1.2	0.4	0.0			
FINNS INARI	56	O	23	12	2	16	3					2	1.683	174
		E	24.4	11.8	1.4	13.3	5.0							
FINNS RISTIINA @	100	O	33	22	6	27	11	1	0	0		1	1.369	174
		E	33.6	24.0	4.3	24.2	13.0	0.6	0.2	0.0				
SWITZERLAND														
SWISS	98	O	37	35	4	14	8					2	1.473	178
		E	38.6	31.0	6.2	14.8	7.4							
U.S.S.R.														
MARIS KOZMODEMYANSK	110	O	43	38	7	13	1	4	4	0	0	3	5.106	174
		E	45.2	36.5	7.4	9.0	4.1	5.1	2.1	0.5	0.1			
MARIS VOLZHSK	101	O	36	45	10	5	2	2	1	0	0	3	0.779	174
		E	38.1	41.7	11.4	4.4	1.8	2.5	1.0	0.1	0.0			
MARIS ZVENIGOVO	103	O	34	43	8	7	4	3	2	2	0	3	2.213	174
		E	35.5	38.0	10.1	7.9	4.6	4.1	2.2	0.5	0.1			

* THE THREE GM(1,3,5,13,14) SAMPLES WERE TESTED FOR GM(15,16,17). TWO WERE NEGATIVE AND ONE WAS POSITIVE FOR ALL THREE.

EXCLUDING ONE GM(1,2,5,13,14,21) AND ONE GM(1,5,13,14,21) SAMPLES.

@ THE ONE GM(1,3,5,13,14) SAMPLE WAS ALSO TESTED AND FOUND POSITIVE FOR GM(15) AND GM(16).

HAPLOTYPES

CAUCASOIDS ASIA INDIA	TOTAL	F / S.E.	3 5 13 14	1 3 21	1 2 21	1 13	REF
IRANIS	106	F	0.646	0.274	0.047	0.033	173
		S.E.	0.033	0.031	0.015	0.012	
EUROPE FINLAND							
ALANDERS ALAND ISLANDS	117	F	0.581	0.297	0.105	0.017	174
		S.E.	0.032	0.030	0.021	0.008	
FINNS INARI	56	F	0.661	0.160	0.179		174
		S.E.	0.045	0.036	0.038		
FINNS RISTIINA	100	F	0.580	0.207	0.208	0.005	174
		S.E.	0.035	0.030	0.030	0.005	
SWITZERLAND							
SWISS	98	F	0.628	0.252	0.120		178
		S.E.	0.035	0.032	0.024		
U.S.S.R.							
MARIS KOZMODEMYANSK	110	F	0.641	0.259	0.064	0.036	174
		S.E.	0.032	0.030	0.017	0.013	
MARIS VOLZHSK	101	F	0.614	0.336	0.035	0.015	174
		S.E.	0.034	0.033	0.013	0.009	
MARIS ZVENIGOVO	103	F	0.587	0.314	0.045	0.034	174
		S.E.	0.034	0.032	0.017	0.013	

TABLE III-13 CONTINUED
TESTED FOR GM 1, 2, 3, 5, 6, 13, 14, 21

CAUCASOIDS

ASIA

INDIA

IRANIS

REF. 173

PHENOTYPES

OBS.	EXP.	
22	20.1	3, 5, 13, 14
14	18.2	1, 3, 5, 13, 14, 21
3	2.5	1, 21
6	5.1	1, 2, 3, 5, 13, 14, 21
2	2.1	1, 2, 21
2	2.5	1, 3, 5, 13, 14
1	0.4	1, 13, 21
0	0.2	1, 2, 13, 21
0	0.0	1, 13
1	0.5	1, 5, 13, 14, 21
0	0.2	1, 2, 5, 13, 14, 21
0	0.1	1, 5, 13, 14
3	1.6	1, 3, 21
0	0.5	1, 2, 3, 21
0	0.1	1, 3, 13, 21
TOTAL 54	54.0	

CHI SQUARE= 2.206   D.F. = 2

HAPLOTYPES

FREQ.	S.E.	
0.610	0.047	3, 5, 13, 14
0.215	0.050	1, 21
0.077	0.026	1, 2, 21
0.018	0.018	1, 13
0.020	0.019	1, 5, 13, 14
0.060	0.037	1, 3, 21

TABLE III-13 CONTINUED
TESTED FOR GM 1, 2, 3, 5, 6, 13, 14, 21

CAUCASOIDS

ASIA

INDIA

PARSIS   REF. 173

PHENOTYPES

OBS.	EXP.	
67	74.7	3, 5, 13, 14
75	65.7	1, 3, 5, 13, 14, 21
8	10.2	1, 21
7	6.5	1, 2, 3, 5, 13, 14, 21
3	2.6	1, 2, 21
63	57.2	1, 3, 5, 13, 14 *
13	13.9	1, 13, 21 #
1	1.7	1, 2, 13, 21
4	4.7	1, 13
4	7.2	1, 5, 13, 14, 21
1	0.9	1, 2, 5, 13, 14, 21
7	6.2	1, 5, 13, 14
4	3.7	1, 3, 21
0	0.4	1, 2, 3, 21
1	2.4	1, 3, 13, 21
TOTAL 258	258.0	

CHI SQUARE= 6.082   D.F. = 8

HAPLOTYPES

FREQ.	S.E.	
0.538	0.022	3, 5, 13, 14
0.199	0.020	1, 21
0.024	0.007	1, 2, 21
0.136	0.019	1, 13
0.071	0.016	1, 5, 13, 14
0.034	0.012	1, 3, 21

* ELEVEN SAMPLES WERE TESTED FOR GM(16,17). ONE WAS GM(16,17); THREE WERE GM(16,17); AND SEVEN WERE GM(-16,-17).

ALL WERE POSITIVE FOR GM(16).

TABLE III-14
TESTED FOR GM 1, 2, 3, 5, 10, 11, 17, 21

PHENOTYPES

CAUCASOIDS EUROPE DENMARK	TOTAL	O./E.	3 5 10 11	1 5 10 11 21	1 3 5 10 11 17 21	1 2 17 21	1 2 3 5 10 11 17 21	1 5 10 11 17	1 2 5 10 11 17 21	1 5 10 11 17	1 2 5 10 11 17	1 2 5 10 11 17	DF	CHI SQ. VALUE	REF.
DANES *	79	O.	34	18	3	11	8	5	0	0	0		3	4.554	131
		E.	32.9	19.3	2.8	13.6	5.4	3.2	0.9	0.7	0.1				
ICELAND ICELANDERS #	66	O.	27	11	3	13	12						2	4.060	98
		E.	23.0	14.5	2.3	17.4	8.8								
YUGOSLAVIA BISTARC	121	O.	85	12	6	6	2	8	0	0	2	0	3	22.828	132
		E.	81.0	21.0	1.4	6.8	1.0	6.5	0.9	0.6	1.6	0.1			
BLJECEVA @	182	O.	131	30	2	8	3	7	0	0	1	0	2	3.209	132
		E.	130.3	31.0	1.8	9.6	1.3	5.9	0.7	0.4	0.8	0.0			
OCEVLGE-VLAHINJE $	137	O.	106	13	3	8	3	3	0	0	4	0	1	2.740	132
		E.	105.1	16.6	0.7	7.0	0.7	2.6	0.6	0.1	3.5	0.1			

HAPLOTYPES

CAUCASOIDS EUROPE DENMARK	TOTAL	F./S.E.	3 5 10 11	1 5 10 11 21	1 2 17 21	1 3 5 10 11 17 21	1 5 10 11 17	1 2 5 10 11 17 21	1 2 5 10 11 17	REF.
DANES	79	F.	0.646	0.189	0.133	0.032	0.032			131
		S.E.	0.038	0.032	0.028	0.014	0.014			
ICELANDERS	66	F.	0.591	0.186	0.224					98
		S.E.	0.043	0.036	0.038					
BISTARC	121	F.	0.818	0.106	0.034	0.033	0.012	0.008	0.006	132
		S.E.	0.025	0.020	0.012	0.012				
BLJECEVA	182	F.	0.846	0.101	0.031	0.019	0.009	0.003	0.003	132
		S.E.	0.019	0.016	0.007	0.007				
OCEVLGE-VLAHINJE	137	F.	0.876	0.069	0.029	0.011	0.010	0.015	0.007	132
		S.E.	0.020	0.015	0.006	0.006				

* EXCLUDING THREE GM(1,2,3,5,10,11,17), THREE GM(3,5,10,11,21), ONE GM(1,2,3,11,17,21), ONE GM(1,3,17,21), AND ONE GM(3,5,10,11,17) SAMPLES.

EXCLUDING ONE GM(1,5,10,11,17,21) AND ONE GM(3,5,10,11,21) SAMPLES.

@ EXCLUDING TWO GM(3,5,10,11,17) SAMPLES.

$ EXCLUDING ONE GM(3,5,10,11,17) SAMPLE.

47

TABLE III-15
TESTED FOR GM 1, 2, 3, 5, 6, 10, 11, 13, 14, 17, 21

PHENOTYPES

CAUCASOIDS

MIDDLE EAST

IRAN

	3 5 10 11 13 14	1 3 5 10 11 13 14 17 21	1 17 17 21	1 2 3 5 10 11 13 14 17 21	1 2 17 21	1 3 5 10 11 14 17	1 3 5 10 11 13 17 21	1 2 10 11 13 17 21	1 3 5 10 11 13 17	1 3 5 10 11 13 14		CHI SQ.	
TOTAL											DF	VALUE	REF.
KURDISTANI * 161 O.	91	34	6	9	4	11	3	0	2	1	3	3.118	8
E.	87.0	38.8	4.3	9.9	2.5	13.3	2.9	0.8	0.5	1.0			

HAPLOTYPES

CAUCASOIDS

MIDDLE EAST

IRAN

	3 5 10 11 13 14	1 3 5 10 11 13 17 21	1 2 17 21	1 3 5 10 11 13 17	1 3 5 10 11 13 14	REF.
TOTAL						
KURDISTANI 161 F.	0.735	0.163	0.042	0.056	0.004	8
S.E.	0.025	0.021	0.011	0.013	0.004	

* EXCLUDING TWO GM(1,3,17,21), ONE GM(1,2,3,5,10,11,13,14,17), ONE GM(1,5,10,11,13,14,17,21), ONE GM(1,3,5,6,10,11,13,14,17,21), AND ONE GM(1,3,5,6,10,11,14,17) SAMPLES.

TABLE III-16.
TESTED FOR GM 1, 2, 3, 5, 6, 11, 13, 15, 16, 17, 21, 24

PHENOTYPES

CAUCASOIDS EUROPE CZECHOSLOVAKIA		3 5 11 13 / 11 13	1 3 5 11 13 17 21 / 17 21	1 17 / 17 21	1 2 3 5 11 13 17 21 / 17 21	1 2 17 / 17 21	1 3 5 11 13 16 17 21 / 16 17	1 3 11 13 15 16 17 21 / 16 17	1 11 13 15 16 17 21 / 16 17	1 11 13 15 16 17 / 16 17	1 2 5 11 13 17 21 / 17 21	1 3 5 11 13 17 21 / 17 21	1 5 11 13 17 21 / 17 21	1 2 5 11 13 16 17 / 16 17	1 5 11 13 15 16 17 / 16 17	1 5 11 13 17 / 17	DF	CHI SQ. VALUE	REF.
TOTAL																			
CENTRAL BOHEMIA *	681	O. 414	139	15	85	18	4	1	0	0	1	4	0	1	0	0	3	0.927	146
		E. 412.5	143.1	12.4	84.1	18.9	3.9	0.7	0.4	0.0	0.7	3.9	0.7	0.4	0.0	0.0			
HUNGARY																			
BUDAPEST #	182	O. 112	43	2	12	5	4	1	0	0	0	1	0	0	0	2	3	5.114	145
		E. 110.8	40.8	3.8	13.8	3.0	3.9	0.7	0.2	0.0	0.2	3.9	0.7	0.2	0.1	0.0			

HAPLOTYPES

CAUCASOIDS EUROPE CZECHOSLOVAKIA		3 5 11 13 17 21	1 3 17 21	1 2 17 21	1 11 13 17	1 11 13 15 16 17	1 5 11 17	REF.
TOTAL								
CENTRAL BOHEMIA	681	F. 0.778	0.135	0.079	0.004	0.004		146
		S.E. 0.011	0.009	0.002	0.002			
HUNGARY								
BUDAPEST	182	F. 0.780	0.144	0.049	0.014	0.014		145
		S.E. 0.022	0.018	0.011	0.006	0.006		

* EXCLUDING ONE GM(1,2,3,5,11,13,17), ONE GM(1,3,17,21), AND ONE GM(3,5,6,11,13) SAMPLES.

EXCLUDING ONE GM(1,2,3,5,11,13,17) AND ONE GM(1,3,17,21) SAMPLES.

TABLE III-17
TESTED FOR GM 1, 2, 3, 5, 6, 10, 11, 13, 15, 16, 17, 21, 23, 24

PHENOTYPES

CAUCASOIDS
EUROPE
ITALY

	3 5 10 11 13 23	3 5 10 11 13	1 3 5 10 11 13 17 21 23	1 3 5 10 11 13 17 21	1 3 5 10 11 13 17 21	1 2 3 5 10 11 13 17 21 23	1 2 3 5 10 11 13 17 21	1 2 17 21
TOTAL								
FERRARA 86 O.	60	0	14	3	1	5	1	2
E.	58.7	0.8	15.2	2.0	1.2	6.1	0.8	1.2

	DF	CHI SQ. VALUE	REF.
	3	1.678	100

HAPLOTYPES

CAUCASOIDS
EUROPE
ITALY

	3 5 10 11 13 23	3 5 10 11 13	1 2 17 21	17 21	REF.
TOTAL					
FERRARA 86 F.	0.737	0.094	0.120	0.048	100
S. E.	0.046	0.038	0.025	0.017	

51

TABLE III-17 CONTINUED
TESTED FOR GM 1, 2, 3, 5, 6, 10, 11, 13, 15, 16, 17, 21, 23, 24

CAUCASOIDS

EUROPE

ITALY

NORTH SARDINIA   REF. 100

PHENOTYPES

OBS.	EXP.	
271	269.0	3, 5, 10, 11, 13, 23
16	18.9	3, 5, 10, 11, 13
62	65.5	1, 3, 5, 10, 11, 13, 17, 21, 23
27	22.5	1, 3, 5, 10, 11, 13, 17, 21
6	6.7	1, 17, 21
6	6.7	1, 2, 3, 5, 10, 11, 13, 17, 21, 23
3	2.3	1, 2, 3, 5, 10, 11, 13, 17, 21
2	1.4	1, 2, 17, 21
15	15.0	1, 3, 5, 10, 11, 13, 17, 23
5	5.2	1, 3, 5, 10, 11, 13, 17
3	3.1	1, 5, 10, 11, 13, 17, 21
0	0.3	1, 2, 5, 10, 11, 13, 17, 21
1	0.4	1, 5, 10, 11, 13, 17
20	19.2	3, 5, 10, 11, 13, 15, 23, 24
3	2.9	1, 3, 5, 10, 11, 13, 15, 17, 21, 23, 24
0	0.3	1, 2, 3, 5, 10, 11, 13, 15, 17, 21, 23, 24
0	0.7	1, 3, 5, 10, 11, 13, 15, 17, 23, 24
1	0.6	1, 3, 5, 10, 11, 13, 15, 16, 17, 23
0	0.2	1, 3, 5, 10, 11, 13, 15, 16, 17
0	0.1	1, 10, 11, 13, 15, 16, 17, 21
0	0.0	1, 2, 10, 11, 13, 15, 16, 17, 21
0	0.0	1, 5, 10, 11, 13, 15, 16, 17, 21
0	0.0	1, 3, 5, 10, 11, 13, 15, 16, 17, 23, 24
0	0.0	1, 10, 11, 13, 15, 16, 17
TOTAL 441	441.0	

CHI SQUARE= 3.248   D.F. = 8

HAPLOTYPES

FREQ.	S.E.	
0.601	0.021	3, 5, 10, 11, 13, 23
0.207	0.019	3, 5, 10, 11, 13
0.123	0.011	1, 17, 21
0.013	0.004	1, 2, 17, 21
0.028	0.006	1, 5, 10, 11, 13, 17
0.026	0.005	3, 5, 10, 11, 13, 15, 23, 24
0.001	0.001	1, 10, 11, 13, 15, 16, 17

TABLE III-17 CONTINUED
TESTED FOR GM 1, 2, 3, 5, 6, 10, 11, 13, 15, 16, 17, 21, 23, 24

CAUCASOIDS

EUROPE

ITALY

NORTHEAST SARDINIA   REF. 100

PHENOTYPES

OBS.	EXP.	
129	126.6	3, 5, 10, 11, 13, 23
9	10.4	3, 5, 10, 11, 13
19	22.3	1, 3, 5, 10, 11, 13, 17, 21, 23
12	8.5	1, 3, 5, 10, 11, 13, 17, 21
2	1.7	1, 17, 21
1	0.6	1, 2, 3, 5, 10, 11, 13, 17, 21, 23
0	0.2	1, 2, 3, 5, 10, 11, 13, 17, 21
0	0.1	1, 2, 17, 21
3	3.6	1, 3, 5, 10, 11, 13, 17, 23
0	1.4	1, 3, 5, 10, 11, 13, 17, 21
0	0.6	1, 5, 10, 11, 13, 15, 17, 21
0	0.0	1, 2, 5, 10, 11, 13, 15, 17, 21
1	0.0	1, 5, 10, 11, 13, 17
19	18.6	3, 5, 10, 11, 13, 15, 23, 24
2	2.0	1, 3, 5, 10, 11, 13, 15, 17, 21, 23, 24
0	0.1	1, 2, 3, 5, 10, 11, 13, 15, 17, 21, 23, 24
0	0.3	1, 3, 5, 10, 11, 13, 15, 17, 23, 24
0	0.6	1, 3, 5, 10, 11, 13, 15, 16, 17, 23
0	0.2	1, 3, 5, 10, 11, 13, 15, 16, 17
0	0.1	1, 10, 11, 13, 15, 16, 17, 21
0	0.0	1, 2, 10, 11, 13, 15, 16, 17, 21
1	0.0	1, 5, 10, 11, 13, 15, 16, 17
0	0.1	1, 3, 5, 10, 11, 13, 15, 16, 17, 23, 24
0	0.0	1, 10, 11, 13, 15, 16, 17
TOTAL 198	198.0	

CHI SQUARE= 4.586   D.F. = 4

HAPLOTYPES

FREQ.	S.E.	
0.602	0.033	3, 5, 10, 11, 13, 23
0.229	0.030	3, 5, 10, 11, 13
0.093	0.015	1, 17, 21
0.003	0.003	1, 2, 17, 21
0.015	0.006	1, 5, 10, 11, 13, 17
0.055	0.012	3, 5, 10, 11, 13, 15, 23, 24
0.003	0.003	1, 10, 11, 13, 15, 16, 17

TABLE III-17   CONTINUED
TESTED FOR GM 1, 2, 3, 5, 6, 10, 11, 13, 15, 16, 17, 21, 23, 24

CAUCASOIDS

EUROPE

ITALY

MOUNTAIN, SARDINIA   REF. 100

PHENOTYPES

OBS.	EXP.	
119	119.0	3, 5, 10, 11, 13, 23
21	20.8	3, 5, 10, 11, 13
28	30.1	1, 3, 5, 10, 11, 13, 17, 21, 23
20	18.9	1, 3, 5, 10, 11, 13, 17, 21
5	4.3	1, 17, 21
4	2.0	1, 2, 3, 5, 10, 11, 13, 17, 21, 23
0	1.3	1, 2, 3, 5, 10, 11, 13, 17, 21
0	0.6	1, 2, 17, 21
2	2.0	1, 3, 5, 10, 11, 13, 17, 23
1	1.3	1, 3, 5, 10, 11, 13, 17
1	0.6	1, 5, 10, 11, 13, 17, 21
0	0.0	1, 2, 5, 10, 11, 13, 17, 21
0	0.0	1, 5, 10, 11, 13, 17
2	1.7	3, 5, 10, 11, 13, 15, 23, 24
0	0.3	1, 3, 5, 10, 11, 13, 15, 17, 21, 23, 24
0	0.0	1, 2, 3, 5, 10, 11, 13, 15, 17, 21, 23, 24
0	0.0	1, 3, 5, 10, 11, 13, 15, 17, 23, 24
TOTAL 203	203.0	

CHI SQUARE= 3.831   D.F. = 5

HAPLOTYPES

FREQ.	S.E.	
0.510	0.030	3, 5, 10, 11, 13, 23
0.320	0.029	3, 5, 10, 11, 13
0.145	0.017	1, 17, 21
0.010	0.005	1, 2, 17, 21
0.010	0.005	1, 5, 10, 11, 13, 17
0.005	0.003	3, 5, 10, 11, 13, 15, 23, 24

TABLE III-17 CONTINUED
TESTED FOR GM 1, 2, 3, 5, 6, 10, 11, 13, 15, 16, 17, 21, 23, 24

CAUCASOIDS

EUROPE

ITALY

SOUTH SARDINIA   REF. 100

PHENOTYPES

OBS.	EXP.	
120	120.5	3, 5, 10, 11, 13, 23
5	5.5	3, 5, 10, 11, 13
24	22.7	1, 3, 5, 10, 11, 13, 17, 21, 23
6	6.0	1, 3, 5, 10, 11, 13, 17, 21
1	1.6	1, 17, 21
1	0.7	1, 2, 3, 5, 10, 11, 13, 17, 21, 23
0	0.2	1, 2, 3, 5, 10, 11, 13, 17, 21
0	0.1	1, 2, 17, 21
5	6.0	1, 3, 5, 10, 11, 13, 17, 23
3	1.6	1, 3, 5, 10, 11, 13, 17
1	0.9	1, 5, 10, 11, 13, 17, 21
0	0.0	1, 2, 5, 10, 11, 13, 17
0	0.1	1, 5, 10, 11, 13, 17
9	8.7	3, 5, 10, 11, 13, 15, 23, 24
1	1.0	1, 3, 5, 10, 11, 13, 15, 17, 21, 23, 24
0	0.0	1, 2, 3, 5, 10, 11, 13, 15, 17, 21, 23, 24
0	0.3	1, 3, 5, 10, 11, 13, 15, 17, 23, 24
TOTAL 176	176.0	

CHI SQUARE= 1.903   D.F. = 4

HAPLOTYPES

FREQ.	S.E.	
0.669	0.034	3, 5, 10, 11, 13, 23
0.177	0.031	3, 5, 10, 11, 13
0.097	0.016	1, 17, 21
0.003	0.003	1, 2, 17, 21
0.026	0.008	1, 5, 10, 11, 13, 17
0.029	0.009	3, 5, 10, 11, 13, 15, 23, 24

TABLE III-17   CONTINUED
TESTED FOR GM 1, 2, 3, 5, 6, 10, 11, 13, 15, 16, 17, 21, 23, 24

CAUCASOIDS

EUROPE

ITALY

SOUTHEAST SARDINIA   REF. 100

PHENOTYPES

OBS.	EXP.	
124	127.2	3, 5, 10, 11, 13, 23
10	9.0	3, 5, 10, 11, 13
22	18.2	1, 3, 5, 10, 11, 13, 17, 21, 23
7	6.3	1, 3, 5, 10, 11, 13, 17, 21
0	1.1	1, 17, 21
9	8.2	1, 3, 5, 10, 11, 13, 17, 23
2	2.8	1, 3, 5, 10, 11, 13, 17
0	1.0	1, 5, 10, 11, 13, 17, 21
0	0.2	1, 5, 10, 11, 13, 17
12	12.3	3, 5, 10, 11, 13, 15, 23, 24
0	1.1	1, 3, 5, 10, 11, 13, 15, 17, 21, 24
2	0.5	1, 3, 5, 10, 11, 13, 15, 17, 23, 24
2	1.3	1, 5, 10, 11, 13, 15, 16, 17, 23
0	0.4	1, 3, 5, 10, 11, 13, 15, 16, 17
0	0.2	1, 10, 11, 13, 15, 16, 17, 21
0	0.1	1, 5, 10, 11, 13, 15, 16, 17
0	0.1	1, 3, 5, 10, 11, 13, 15, 16, 17, 23, 24
0	0.0	1, 10, 11, 13, 15, 16, 17
TOTAL 190	190.0	

CHI SQUARE= 5.211   D.F. = 5

HAPLOTYPES

FREQ.	S.E.	
0.629	0.033	3, 5, 10, 11, 13, 23
0.218	0.031	3, 5, 10, 11, 13
0.076	0.014	1, 17, 21
0.034	0.009	1, 5, 10, 11, 13, 17
0.038	0.010	3, 5, 10, 11, 13, 15, 23, 24
0.005	0.004	1, 10, 11, 13, 15, 16, 17

TABLE III-17 CONTINUED
TESTED FOR GM 1, 2, 3, 5, 6, 10, 11, 13, 15, 16, 17, 21, 23, 24

CAUCASOIDS

EUROPE

NETHERLANDS

DUTCH

PHENOTYPES *   REF. 31

OBS.	EXP.	
344	340.6	3, 5, 10, 11, 13, 23
50	49.0	3, 5, 10, 11, 13
126	133.1	1, 3, 5, 10, 11, 13, 17, 21, 23
66	73.1	1, 3, 5, 10, 11, 13, 17, 21
36	27.3	1, 17, 21
72	72.4	1, 2, 3, 5, 10, 11, 13, 17, 21, 23
45	39.8	1, 2, 3, 5, 10, 11, 13, 17, 21
34	37.8	1, 2, 17, 21
4	2.7	1, 3, 5, 10, 11, 13, 17, 23
0	1.5	1, 3, 5, 10, 11, 13, 17
1	1.1	1, 3, 5, 10, 11, 13, 17, 21
1	0.6	1, 2, 5, 10, 11, 13, 17, 21
0	0.0	1, 5, 10, 11, 13, 17
4	2.7	3, 5, 6, 10, 11, 13, 23, 24
1	1.5	3, 5, 6, 10, 11, 13, 24
1	1.1	1, 3, 5, 6, 11, 17, 21, 24
0	0.6	1, 2, 3, 5, 6, 11, 17, 21, 24
0	0.0	1, 3, 5, 6, 10, 11, 13, 17, 21, 24
0	0.0	3, 5, 6, 11, 24
TOTAL 785	785.0	

CHI SQUARE= 7.902   D.F. = 9

HAPLOTYPES

FREQ.	S.E.	
0.455	0.014	3, 5, 10, 11, 13, 23
0.250	0.013	3, 5, 10, 11, 13
0.186	0.010	1, 17, 21
0.101	0.008	1, 2, 17, 21
0.004	0.002	1, 5, 10, 11, 13, 17
0.004	0.002	3, 5, 6, 11, 24

* EXCLUDING ONE GM(1,3,17,21), ONE GM(3,5,10,11,13,21,23), ONE GM(3,5,10,11,13,21,23), ONE GM(1,2,5,10,11,13,17,21,23), ONE GM(1,3,5,11,17,21,23,24), ONE GM(3,5,10,11,13,23,24), ONE GM(1,3,5,10,11,13,15,17,21,23), ONE GM(1,2,17,21,23), ONE GM(1,10,11,13,15,16,17,21), ONE GM(1,3,5,10,11,13,23), ONE GM(1,3,5,10,11,13,15,16,17,23), TWO GM(1,2,3,5,10,11,13,17,23), AND ONE GM(1,5,6,10,11,13,17,21,23) SAMPLES.

TABLE III-18
TESTED FOR GM 1, 2, 5

PHENOTYPES

Population	TOTAL		5	1 5	1	1 2 5	1 2	DF	CHI SQ. VALUE
CAUCASOIDS-ARABS									
AFRICA									
ALGERIA									
ALH-AZZI TIDIKELT	80	O.	1	75	2	2	0	0	
		E.	1.0	75.2	1.8	1.7	0.3		
HARRATIN TIDIKELT	304	O.	24	251	19	6	4	1	0.955
		E.	23.9	250.2	19.8	7.4	2.7		
CHAAMBAS	224	O.	51	134	17	18	4	1	1.538
		E.	51.5	135.2	15.5	15.3	6.4		
M'SIRDAS	240	O.	71	149	16	4	0	1	1.427
		E.	71.2	149.4	15.4	3.0	1.0		
REGUIBAT	297	O.	59	184	35	12	7	1	0.001
		E.	59.0	184.0	35.0	12.1	6.9		
REGUIBAT TINDOUF	333	O.	67	208	40	11	7	1	0.041
		E.	66.9	207.8	40.3	11.4	6.6		
TADJAKANT TINDOUF	59	O.	8	41	5	3	2	1	0.133
		E.	8.0	40.8	5.2	3.4	1.6		
HOGGAR MTS.	144	O.	5	121	13	5	0	1	2.250
		E.	5.0	122.0	12.1	3.5	1.5		
TOUREG AIR PLATEAU	66	O.	6	55	3	1	1	0	
		E.	6.0	54.7	3.3	1.5	0.5		
TOUREG HOGGAR MTS.	56	O.	3	44	4	4	1	1	0.209
		E.	3.0	44.3	3.7	3.5	1.4		
LIBYA									
TRIPOLIS AND BENGHASI	168	O.	48	89	15	12	4	1	0.440
		E.	48.3	89.5	14.3	10.8	5.2		

HAPLOTYPES

Population		5	1	1 2	1 5	REF.
ALH-AZZI TIDIKELT	F.	0.112	0.151	0.012	0.725	23
	S.E.	0.056	0.054	0.009	0.077	
HARRATIN TIDIKELT	F.	0.281	0.255	0.017	0.447	23
	S.E.	0.028	0.027	0.005	0.037	
CHAAMBAS	F.	0.479	0.263	0.050	0.208	133
	S.E.	0.029	0.031	0.010	0.038	
M'SIRDAS	F.	0.545	0.253	0.008	0.194	133
	S.E.	0.027	0.031	0.004	0.037	
REGUIBAT	F.	0.446	0.343	0.033	0.178	133
	S.E.	0.026	0.026	0.007	0.033	
REGUIBAT TINDOUF	F.	0.448	0.348	0.027	0.177	123
	S.E.	0.024	0.025	0.006	0.031	
TADJAKANT TINDOUF	F.	0.367	0.298	0.044	0.292	123
	S.E.	0.060	0.060	0.019	0.079	
HOGGAR MTS.	F.	0.187	0.289	0.017	0.506	6
	S.E.	0.041	0.039	0.008	0.055	
TOUREG AIR PLATEAU	F.	0.301	0.224	0.015	0.460	6
	S.E.	0.059	0.059	0.011	0.080	
TOUREG HOGGAR MTS.	F.	0.232	0.258	0.045	0.464	6
	S.E.	0.065	0.061	0.020	0.087	
TRIPOLIS AND BENGHASI	F.	0.536	0.292	0.049	0.124	195
	S.E.	0.032	0.035	0.012	0.042	

TABLE III-18 CONTINUED
TESTED FOR GM 1,2,5

PHENOTYPES

CAUCASOIDS-ARABS

MIDDLE EAST

JORDAN	TOTAL		5	1 5	5 1	1 2 5	1 2	CHI SQ DF	VALUE
BEDOUINS	285	O.	117	130	14	21	3	1	1.844
		E.	117.8	130.9	12.5	18.2	5.6		
JORDANIANS	179	O.	68	93	7	9	2	1	0.073
		E.	68.1	93.1	6.8	8.6	2.3		
PALESTINIANS	73	O.	30	34	1	7	1	0	
		E.	30.0	34.1	0.9	6.8	1.2		
LEBANON									
CHRISTIANS									
ARMENIAN ORTHODOX	55	O.	31	16	5	1	2	1	1.663
		E.	28.4	20.0	3.5	2.2	0.8		
GREEK CATHOLIC	134	O.	65	47	12	9	1	2	2.562
		E.	64.5	49.9	9.7	7.0	2.9		
GREEK ORTHODOX	125	O.	68	43	5	7	2	2	0.330
		E.	69.2	40.8	6.0	6.8	2.2		
MARONITES	587	O.	285	204	46	45	7	2	7.447
		E.	285.7	211.0	39.0	36.7	14.7		
ʹ OMITTING GM(2)	587	O.	285	249	53			1	0.017
		E.	285.7	247.7	53.7				

HAPLOTYPES

		5	1	1 2	1 5	REF.
BEDOUINS	F.	0.643	0.209	0.043	0.105	180
	S.E.	0.023	0.027	0.009	0.032	
JORDANIANS	F.	0.617	0.195	0.031	0.157	180
	S.E.	0.029	0.035	0.009	0.042	
PALESTINIANS	F.	0.642	0.113	0.056	0.190	180
	S.E.	0.045	0.053	0.019	0.064	
ARMENIAN ORTHODOX	F.	0.718	0.254	0.028	0.016	135
	S.E.	0.043	0.042	0.016		
GREEK CATHOLIC	F.	0.694	0.268	0.038	0.012	135
	S.E.	0.028	0.027	0.012		
GREEK ORTHODOX	F.	0.744	0.219	0.037	0.012	135
	S.E.	0.028	0.026	0.012		
MARONITES	F.	0.698	0.258	0.045	0.006	135
	S.E.	0.013	0.013	0.006		
OMITTING GM(2)	F.	0.698	0.302			
	S.E.	0.013	0.013			

TABLE III-18 CONTINUED
TESTED FOR GM 1,2,5

CAUCASOIDS-ARABS
MIDDLE EAST
LEBANON
MOSLEMS

PHENOTYPES

		TOTAL	5	1/5	1	1/2/5	1/2	CHI SQ. DF	CHI SQ. VALUE
CHIITE	O.	257	132	89	15	18	3	2	1.644
	E.		133.9	87.9	14.4	15.3	5.5		
DRUZE	O.	107	37	53	9	7	1	2	4.748
	E.		42.0	45.1	12.1	5.0	2.9		
SUNNITE	O.	293	135	132	13	11	2	1	0.356
	E.		135.3	132.3	12.5	10.1	2.9		

HAPLOTYPES

		5	1	1/2	1/5	REF.
CHIITE	F.	0.722	0.237	0.041		135
	S.E.	0.020	0.019	0.009		
DRUZE	F.	0.626	0.336	0.038		135
	S.E.	0.033	0.032	0.013		
SUNNITE	F.	0.679	0.207	0.022	0.092	135
	S.E.	0.021	0.028	0.006	0.031	

TABLE III-19
TESTED FOR GM 1,2,3,5

CAUCASOIDS-ARABS
AFRICA
EGYPT

PHENOTYPES

		TOTAL	3/5	1/3/5	1/2/3/5	1/3	1/2	1/5	1/2/5	DF	VALUE
ARABS	O.	69	27	32	3	1	0	4	2	2	1.954
	E.		27.4	30.3	2.6	1.9	0.6	5.8	0.5		

HAPLOTYPES

		3/5	1	1/2	1/5	REF.
ARABS	F.	0.630	0.192	0.022	0.155	45
	S.E.	0.041	0.053	0.012	0.051	

TABLE III-20
TESTED FOR GM 1, 2, 3, 5, 10, 11

PHENOTYPES

		3 5 10 11	1 3 5 10 11	1	1 2 3 5 10 11	1 3 10 11	1 2 3 10 11	1 5 10 11	1 2 5 10 11	CHI SQ. DF	VALUE	REF.
CAUCASOIDS-ARABS												
AFRICA												
EGYPT	TOTAL											
SINAI												
BEDUIN JEBELIYA	63 O.	6	32	4				21		1	0.870	11
	E.	7.7	28.6	4.3				22.4				
BEDUIN TOWARA	163 O.	46	82	8	3	0	1	16	0	3	3.324	11
	E.	50.2	74.3	9.5	2.9	1.0	0.1	17.0	1.8			

HAPLOTYPES

		3 5 10 11	1	1 2	1 3 10 11	1 5 10 11	REF.
ARABS							
AFRICA							
EGYPT	TOTAL						
SINAI							
BEDUIN JEBELIYA	63 F.	0.349	0.260			0.390	11
	S.E.	0.042	0.060			0.063	
BEDUIN TOWARA	163 F.	0.555	0.241	0.034	0.013	0.157	11
	S.E.	0.028	0.034	0.010	0.012	0.031	

TABLE III-21
TESTED FOR GM 1, 2, 3, 5, 10, 11, 13, 14, 17, 21, 23

CAUCASOIDS-GYPSIES

EUROPE   REF. 20

PHENOTYPES

OBS.	EXP.	
53	55.3	3, 5, 10, 11, 13, 14, 23
9	5.9	3, 5, 10, 11, 13, 14
40	41.0	1, 3, 5, 10, 11, 13, 14, 17, 21, 23
6	11.6	1, 3, 5, 10, 11, 13, 14, 17, 21
9	5.2	1, 17, 21
2	1.1	1, 17, 21, 23
12	10.3	1, 2, 3, 5, 10, 11, 13, 14, 17, 21, 23
2	3.3	1, 2, 3, 5, 10, 11, 13, 14, 17, 21
4	3.4	1, 2, 17, 21
0	0.3	1, 2, 17, 21, 23
31	24.4	1, 3, 5, 10, 11, 13, 14, 17, 23
5	4.1	1, 3, 5, 10, 11, 13, 14, 17
1	1.2	1, 5, 10, 11, 13, 14, 17, 21
0	0.1	1, 5, 10, 11, 13, 14, 17, 21, 23
0	0.3	1, 2, 5, 10, 11, 13, 14, 17
0	0.4	1, 5, 10, 11, 13, 14, 17
46	48.0	1, 3, 5, 10, 11, 13, 14, 23
1	0.7	1, 3, 5, 10, 11, 13, 14
2	2.5	1, 10, 11, 13, 17, 21
1	3.0	1, 10, 11, 13, 17, 21, 23
0	0.7	1, 2, 10, 11, 13, 17, 21
1	0.7	1, 2, 10, 11, 13, 17, 21, 23
0	0.3	1, 5, 10, 11, 13, 14, 17
0	0.3	1, 10, 11, 13, 17, 23
0	0.9	1, 10, 11, 13, 17, 23
1	0.7	1, 2, 3, 5, 10, 11, 13, 14, 17, 23
0	0.2	1, 2, 5, 10, 11, 13, 14, 17, 21, 23
0	0.1	1, 2, 5, 10, 11, 13, 14, 17, 23
TOTAL 226	226.0	

CHI SQUARE=14.236   D.F. = 8

HAPLOTYPES

FREQ.	S.E.	
0.359	0.032	3, 5, 10, 11, 13, 14, 23
0.161	0.026	3, 5, 10, 11, 13, 14
0.151	0.020	1, 17, 21
0.016	0.012	1, 17, 21, 23
0.043	0.010	1, 2, 17, 21
0.018	0.011	1, 5, 10, 11, 13, 14, 17
0.168	0.024	1, 3, 5, 10, 11, 13, 14, 23
0.009	0.011	1, 3, 5, 10, 11, 13, 14
0.037	0.013	1, 10, 11, 13, 17, 23
0.037	0.014	1, 10, 11, 13, 17
0.002	0.002	1, 2, 5, 10, 11, 13, 14, 17, 23

TABLE III-22
TESTED FOR GM 1, 2, 5

PHENOTYPES

CAUCASOIDS-JEWS

AFRICA

MOROCCO

	TOTAL		5	1 5	1	1 2 5	1 2	CHI SQ. DF	VALUE
JEWS	181	O.	77	89	8	6	1		
		E.	77.2	89.2	7.7	5.5	1.5	1	0.246

MIDDLE EAST

IRAN

	TOTAL		5	1 5	1	1 2 5	1 2	CHI SQ. DF	VALUE
JEWS	142	O.	83	48	2	9	0		
		E.	83.4	48.2	1.5	7.8	1.1	1	1.434

HAPLOTYPES

		5	1	1 2	1 5	REF.
	F.	0.653	0.206	0.019	0.121	126
	S.E.	0.028	0.035	0.007	0.041	
	F.	0.766	0.102	0.032	0.100	126
	S.E.	0.027	0.039	0.010	0.044	

63

TABLE III-23
TESTED FOR GM 1, 2, 3, 5, 10, 11

PHENOTYPES

CAUCASOIDS-JEWS
MIDDLE EAST
ISRAEL

	TOTAL	3 5 10 11	1 3 5 10 11	1	1 2 3 5 10 11	1 2 10 11	1 10 11	1 2 5 10 11	1 5 10 11	1 2 5 10 11	1 3	DF	CHI SQ. VALUE	REF.
KURDISH JEWS	88	O.	52	33	1					1		1	1	0.345	41
		E.	52.9	31.2	1.1					1.4		1.4			
YEMENITE JEWS	75	O.	33	28	7	1	0	1	0	3	2		1	3.509	41
		E.	30.1	32.9	4.7	1.9	0.8	0.7	0.1	3.6	0.2				

HAPLOTYPES

CAUCASOIDS-JEWS
MIDDLE EAST
ISRAEL

	TOTAL	3 5 10 11	1	1 2	1 10 11	1 5 10 11	1 3	REF.
KURDISH JEWS	88	F.	0.775	0.113			0.056	0.056	41
		S.E.	0.032	0.052			0.039	0.039	
YEMENITE JEWS	75	F.	0.633	0.252	0.020	0.017	0.078		41
		S.E.	0.039	0.048	0.011	0.020	0.036		

TABLE III-24
TESTED FOR GM 1, 2, 3, 5, 6, 13, 14, 15, 16, 21 *

PHENOTYPES

CAUCASOIDS-JEWS
N. AMERICA
U.S.A.

Phenotype (GM factors)	ASHKENAZIC JEWS 248 O.	E.
1 3 5 13 14 21	156	158.1
1 2 3 5 13 14 21	58	54.5
1 3 5 13 14 21	3	4.7
1 2 3 5 13 14 21	17	18.1
1 3 5 13 14 15 16 21	5	3.6
1 3 5 13 15 16 21	4	3.2
1 3 5 13 15 16 21	0	0.6
1 2 13 15 16 21	0	0.2
1 3 5 13 15 16 21	0	0.0
1 5 13 14 21	5	4.0
1 2 5 13 14 21	0	0.7
1 5 13 14 15 16	0	0.2
1 5 13 13 14	0	0.0
1 5 13 13 14	0	0.0

	DF	CHI SQ. VALUE	REF.
	3	2.740	171

HAPLOTYPES

CAUCASOIDS-JEWS
N. AMERICA
U.S.A.

Haplotype (GM factors)	3 5 13 14 21	1 3 5 13 14 21	1 2 3 5 13 16 21	1 13 15 16	1 5 13 14	REF.
ASHKENAZIC JEWS 248 F.	0.798	0.138	0.046	0.008	0.010	171
S.E.	0.018	0.016	0.009	0.004	0.004	

* ONLY GM(1,-21) SAMPLES WERE TESTED FOR GM(15) AND GM(16).

TABLE IV-1
TESTED FOR GM 1, 2, 3, 5, 6, 13, 14

KHOISAN-KHOIKHOI

AFRICA

S. W. AFRICA

TOPNAAR, KUISEB VALLEY   REF.   63

PHENOTYPES

OBS.	EXP.	
16	15.6	1, 5, 13, 14
5	4.6	1, 13
23	20.7	1, 5, 6, 13, 14
5	5.9	1, 5, 6, 14
1	1.4	1, 5, 6, 13
0	0.1	1, 5, 6
0	1.2	1, 2, 5, 13, 14
0	1.1	1, 2, 13
2	1.1	1, 2, 5, 6, 14
1	0.2	1, 2, 5, 6
0	0.1	1, 2
2	3.0	1, 3, 5, 13, 14
0	1.6	1, 3, 5, 6, 13, 14
1	0.2	1, 2, 3, 5, 13, 14
1	0.1	3, 5, 13, 14
TOTAL 57	57.0	

CHI SQUARE=10.863   D.F. = 4

HAPLOTYPES

FREQ.	S.E.	
0.311	0.060	1, 5, 13, 14
0.285	0.059	1, 13
0.282	0.048	1, 5, 6, 14
0.042	0.030	1, 5, 6
0.035	0.017	1, 2
0.044	0.019	3, 5, 13, 14

TABLE IV-2
TESTED FOR GM 1, 2, 3, 5, 6, 13, 14, 21

PHENOTYPES

KHOISAN-KHOIKHOI

AFRICA

S.W. AFRICA

		1 5 13 14	1 3 13 14	1 5 6 13 14	1 5 6 13	1 5 6 13	1 5 6 21	1 2 5 13 14 21	1 2 13 21	1 2 5 6 14 21	1 2 5 6 21	1 2 21	CHI SQ. DF	CHI SQ. VALUE	REF.
SESFONTEIN	TOTAL 42												2	0.998	175
	O.	20	4	12	1	1	0	1	2	1	0	0			
	E.	19.7	4.7	11.4	1.5	0.8	0.0	1.7	1.3	0.7	0.1	0.1			

HAPLOTYPES

KHOISAN-KHOIKHOI

AFRICA

S.W. AFRICA

		1 5 13 14	1 13 14	1 5 6 14	1 5 6 14	1 5 6 21	1 2 21	REF.
SESFONTEIN	TOTAL 42							175
	F.	0.429	0.333	0.163	0.027	0.027	0.048	
	S.E.	0.071	0.069	0.045	0.027	0.027	0.023	

67

TABLE IV-3
TESTED FOR GM 1, 2, 3, 5, 6, 13, 14, 21

KHOISAN-MIXED

AFRICA

S. W. AFRICA

KEETMANSHOOP   REF. 175

PHENOTYPES

OBS.	EXP.	
86	91.3	1, 5, 13, 14
18	14.0	1, 13
5	4.3	1, 5, 6, 13, 14
0	1.2	1, 5, 6, 14
1	0.6	1, 5, 6, 13
0	0.0	1, 5, 6
0	0.8	1, 2, 5, 13, 14, 21
1	0.6	1, 2, 13, 21
0	0.0	1, 2, 5, 6, 14, 21
0	0.0	1, 2, 5, 6, 21
1	0.2	1, 2, 21
19	12.9	1, 5, 13, 14, 21
4	10.1	1, 13, 21
1	0.6	1, 5, 6, 14, 21
0	0.2	1, 5, 6, 21
0	1.8	1, 21
0	0.3	1, 2, 5, 14, 21
8	5.2	1, 5, 14, 21
4	3.7	1, 5, 14
1	0.9	1, 3, 5, 13, 14
0	0.0	1, 3, 5, 6, 13, 14
0	0.0	1, 2, 3, 5, 13, 14, 21
0	0.1	1, 3, 5, 13, 14, 21
0	0.0	3, 5, 13, 14

TOTAL 149   149.0

CHI SQUARE= 13.618   D.F. = 4

HAPLOTYPES

FREQ.	S.E.	
0.391	0.044	1, 5, 13, 14
0.307	0.035	1, 13
0.017	0.009	1, 5, 6, 14
0.006	0.007	1, 5, 6
0.007	0.005	1, 2, 21
0.111	0.018	1, 21
0.158	0.032	1, 5, 14
0.003	0.003	3, 5, 13, 14

TABLE IV-4
TESTED FOR GM 1, 2, 3, 5, 6, 13, 14

PHENOTYPES

KHOISAN-SAN

AFRICA

BOTSWANA

	TOTAL	1 5 13 14	1 3	1	1 5 6 13 14	1 5 6 14	1 5 6 13	1 5 6	1 5 13	1 5	DF	CHI SQ. VALUE	REF.
CENTRAL-SOUTH KALAHARI DES.	112	O. 57	38	4	5	2	0	2	1	3	2	2.812	62
		E. 56.9	36.0	5.8	5.3	1.8	1.2	0.8	2.6	1.6			
MAINLY SOUTHERN	72	O. 30	23	2	14	2	1	0			0		64
		E. 30.6	23.5	1.3	12.4	3.2	0.7	0.2					

HAPLOTYPES

KHOISAN-SAN

AFRICA

BOTSWANA

	TOTAL	1 5 13 14	1 3	1	1 5 6 14	1 5 6	1 5	REF.
CENTRAL-SOUTH KALAHARI DES.	112	F. 0.317	0.384	0.227	0.028	0.014	0.030	62
		S.E. 0.035	0.047	0.043	0.012	0.010	0.014	
MAINLY SOUTHERN	72	F. 0.290	0.452	0.135	0.111	0.012		64
		S.E. 0.044	0.062	0.050	0.028	0.012		

TABLE IV-5
TESTED FOR GM 1, 2, 3, 5, 6, 13, 14, 21

PHENOTYPES

KHOISAN-SAN — AFRICA — BOTSWANA

Population	Total		1,5,13,14	1,13	1,13,14,21	1,13,21	1,5,6,13,14	1,5,6,14,21	1,5,6,13	1,5,6,14	1,5,13,21	1,5,6,21	1,5	DF	CHI SQ. VALUE	REF.
!KUNG /AI/AI	62	O.	33	16	4	5	2	2		0			0	1	1.216	175
		E.	32.4	15.5	4.9	6.5	1.8	1.8		0.2			0.0			
!KUNG /DU/DA	100	O.	38	33	11	11	1	6		0			0	2	3.869	175
		E.	41.5	30.8	7.1	13.3	1.4	5.1		0.7			0.1			
NARON GHANZI	138	O.	46	40	14	18	1	13	2	0	1	1	0	3	3.246	175
		E.	49.6	38.1	10.0	19.5	2.5	12.1	1.8	0.6	2.2	0.7	0.2			

HAPLOTYPES

KHOISAN-SAN — AFRICA — BOTSWANA

Population	Total		1,5,13,14	1,13	1,5,6,14	1,5,6	1,5	1	REF.
!KUNG /AI/AI	62	F.	0.378	0.501	0.105		0.016		175
		S.E.	0.050	0.051	0.028		0.011		
!KUNG /DU/DA	100	F.	0.295	0.555	0.120		0.030		175
		S.E.	0.036	0.039	0.023		0.012		
NARON GHANZI	138	F.	0.270	0.526	0.134	0.050	0.015	0.005	175
		S.E.	0.030	0.033	0.021	0.014	0.009	0.005	

TABLE IV-5 CONTINUED
TESTED FOR GM 1, 2, 3, 5, 6, 13, 14, 21

PHENOTYPES

KHOISAN-SAN
AFRICA
BOTSWANA

	TOTAL	1 5 13 14	1 13	1 13 21	1 5 14 21	1 5 6 13 14	1 5 6 14	1 5 6 13	1 5 6 21	1 5 6	1 5 6 13 14 21	DF	CHI SQ. VALUE	REF.
!KUNG DOBE	394													
O.		155	142	33	40	19	2							
E.		156.0	143.1	32.1	38.6	17.5	2.6	1.6	0	2	0	0	0	2	1.340	175
E.		164.4	135.9	22.3	45.8	17.5	3.9	1.9	0.3	1.7	0.3	0.0	0.4	3	8.180	

HAPLOTYPES

KHOISAN-SAN
AFRICA
BOTSWANA

	TOTAL	1 5 13 14	1 13	1 13 21	1 5 6 14	1 5 13 14 21	REF.
!KUNG DOBE	394						
F.		0.269	0.603	0.081	0.024	0.004 0.020	175
S.E.		0.018	0.020	0.011	0.006	0.003 0.008	
F.		0.286	0.587	0.099	0.024	0.004	
S.E.		0.018	0.019	0.011	0.006	0.003	

TABLE IV-5 CONTINUED
TESTED FOR GM 1, 2, 3, 5, 6, 13, 14, 21

PHENOTYPES

KHOISAN-SAN
AFRICA
BOTSWANA

	TOTAL	1 5 13 14	1 13 21	1 5 13 14 21	1 13 21	1 5 6 14 21	1 5 6 13 14	1 5 6 14	1 5 13	1 5 21	1 5	1 5 6 13 14 21	DF	CHI SQ. VALUE	REF.
!KUNG NORTHERN	100														
O.		26	13	30	12	12	4	2	1	0	0				
E.		27.6	13.3	27.6	12.4	10.2	2.9	2.7	0.6	0.3	0.0	0	3	3.459	175
E.		35.3	9.2	18.0	15.1	10.6	6.2	4.0	0.4	0.3	0.0	1.7	3	15.911	

HAPLOTYPES

KHOISAN-SAN
AFRICA
BOTSWANA

	TOTAL	1 5 13 14	1 13 21	1 5 6 14	1 5 21	1 5	1 5 13 14 21	REF.
!KUNG NORTHERN	100							
F.		0.272	0.365	0.170	0.080	0.008	0.106	175
S.E.		0.043	0.043	0.033	0.019	0.008	0.031	
F.		0.360	0.303	0.250	0.080	0.007		
S.E.		0.039	0.038	0.031	0.019	0.008		

TABLE IV-5   CONTINUED
TESTED FOR GM 1,2,3,5,6,13,14,21

PHENOTYPES

KHOISAN-SAN

AFRICA

S.W. AFRICA

		1 5 13 14	1 13	1 5 13 14 21	1 13 21	1 5 6 13 14	1 5 6 14	1 5 6 13	1 5 6 21	1 5 6	1 5 14 21	1 5 14	DF	CHI SQ. VALUE	REF.
!KUNG TSUMKWE	197														
	O.	77	74	13	17	1	0	6	0	0	4	0	4	11.313	175
	E.	79.4	69.4	10.0	26.1	1.6	0.3	4.2	0.8	0.1	2.2	0.5			

HAPLOTYPES

KHOISAN-SAN

AFRICA

S.W. AFRICA

		1 5 13 14	1 13	1 13 21	1 5 6	1 5 14	REF.
!KUNG TSUMKWE	197						
	F.	0.227	0.593	0.117	0.018	0.050	175
	S.F.	0.031	0.027	0.016	0.007	0.022	

73

TABLE IV-5 CONTINUED
TESTED FOR GM 1, 7, 8, 5, 6, 13, 14, 21

KHOISAN-SAN

AFRICA

BOTSWANA

!KUNG, NGAMI   REF. 175

PHENOTYPES

OBS.	EXP.	
52	52.6	1, 5, 13, 14
32	36.3	1, 13
20	19.3	1, 5, 13, 14, 21
28	18.8	1, 13, 21
2	2.4	1, 21
6	5.5	1, 5, 6, 13, 14
0	0.7	1, 5, 6, 14, 21
1	0.5	1, 5, 6, 14
3	2.1	1, 5, 6, 13
0	0.6	1, 5, 6, 21
0	0.3	1, 5, 6
13	9.4	1, 5, 13
0	2.4	1, 5, 21
0	0.6	1, 5
0	0.3	1, 5, 6, 13, 14, 21

TOTAL 152   152.0

CHI SQUARE= 6.611   D.F. = 4

HAPLOTYPES

FREQ.	S.E.	
0.254	0.030	1, 5, 13, 14
0.489	0.033	1, 13
0.126	0.022	1, 21
0.019	0.009	1, 5, 6, 14
0.014	0.008	1, 5, 6
0.063	0.017	1, 5, 13, 14, 21
0.033	0.016	1, 5, 13, 14, 21

TABLE IV-5 CONTINUED
TESTED FOR GM 1, 2, 3, 5, 6, 13, 14, 21

KHOISAN-SAN

AFRICA

BOTSWANA

KAUKAU, GHANZI   REF. 175

PHENOTYPES

OBS.	EXP.	
86	88.3	1, 5, 13, 14
67	64.3	1, 13
29	27.6	1, 5, 13, 14, 21
44	40.2	1, 13, 21
6	6.3	1, 21
21	16.8	1, 5, 6, 13, 14
0	3.3	1, 5, 6, 14, 21
1	1.3	1, 5, 6, 14
0	1.6	1, 5, 6, 13
1	0.5	1, 5, 6, 21
1	0.1	1, 5, 6
7	5.6	1, 5, 13
0	1.7	1, 5, 21
0	0.1	1, 5
0	0.4	1, 5, 6, 13, 14, 21
1	0.7	1, 5, 14, 21
0	0.1	1, 5, 14
TOTAL 259	259.0	

CHI SQUARE= 9.221   D.F. = 4

HAPLOTYPES

FREQ.	S.E.	
0.253	0.025	1, 5, 13, 14
0.498	0.025	1, 13
0.156	0.018	1, 21
0.041	0.009	1, 5, 6, 14
0.006	0.004	1, 5, 6
0.022	0.008	1, 5
0.015	0.011	1, 5, 13, 14, 21
0.009	0.009	1, 5, 14

TABLE V-1
TESTED FOR GM 1, 2, 3, 5, 6, 13, 14, 21

PHENOTYPES

LAPPS
EUROPE
FINLAND

	TOTAL		3 5 13 14	1 3 5 13 14 21	14 21	1 2 3 5 13 14 21	1 3 5 13 14	1 2 13 14 21	1 5 13 14	1 3 13 21	1 2 13 21	1 13	DF	CHI SQ. VALUE	REF.
FISHER	254	O.	52	113	64	10	3	12	3	0	0	0			
		E.	52.1	114.3	62.7	10.2	1.4	11.7	1.4			0.1	3	3.043	174
		E.	50.5	115.8	62.7	10.3	2.9	11.7	2.9	1.5	0.1	0.0	2	0.158	
MOUNTAIN	132	O.	56	36	13	16	1	10	1	0	0	0			
		E.	51.6	44.0	9.4	17.3	0.6	8.8	0.6			0.1	1	3.467	174
		E.	51.3	44.2	9.4	17.4	0.9	8.8	0.9	0.3	0.1	0.0	1	3.647	
NELLIM SKOLT	153	O.	86	45	3	9	5	1		3	1	0			
		E.	87.2	41.5	4.9	8.4	6.8	2.2		1.6	0.3	0.1	3	4.032	174
SEVETTIJARVI SKOLT	345	O.	142	148	15	8	23	2	2	6	1	0			
		E.	151.3	127.6	25.1	7.6	24.5	3.1	3.1	5.3	0.3	0.3	2	8.215	174
		E.	155.3	124.8	25.1	7.4	20.1	3.1	3.1	8.1	0.5	0.7	4	10.885	
		E.	142.0	148.0	15.0	8.2	23.0	2.4	2.4	5.6	0.4	0.5	1	0.074	
		E.	142.9	148.0	14.5	8.1	21.2	2.4	2.4	6.7	0.5	0.8	3	0.393	

HAPLOTYPES

LAPPS
EUROPE

FINLAND	TOTAL		3 5 13 14	1 21	1 2 21	1 13	1 3 5 13 14	1 3 5 13 14 21	REF.
FISHER	254	F.	0.453	0.497	0.044	0.006			174
		S.E.	0.022	0.022	0.009	0.003			
		F.	0.446	0.497	0.044		0.013		
		S.E.	0.023	0.022	0.009		0.007		
MOUNTAIN	132	F.	0.625	0.267	0.105	0.004			174
		S.E.	0.030	0.028	0.019	0.004			
		F.	0.623	0.267	0.105		0.006		
		S.E.	0.030	0.028	0.019		0.006		
NELLIM SKOLT	153	F.	0.755	0.179	0.036	0.029			174
		S.E.	0.025	0.022	0.011	0.010			
SEVETTIJARVI SKOLT	345	F.	0.662	0.269	0.016	0.028	0.024		174
		S.E.	0.019	0.017	0.005	0.011	0.014		
		F.	0.671	0.269	0.016	0.043			
		S.E.	0.018	0.017	0.005	0.008			
		F.	0.641	0.209	0.016	0.039	0.013	0.083	
		S.E.	0.021	0.025	0.005	0.014	0.017	0.028	
		F.	0.644	0.205	0.016	0.048		0.088	
		S.E.	0.020	0.025	0.005	0.009		0.027	

77

TABLE VI-1
TESTED FOR GM 1, 2, 5, 6

PHENOTYPES

MELANESIANS

OCEANIA

PAP. N. GUINEA

	TOTAL	1 5 1	1	1 2 5	1 2	DF	CHI SQ. VALUE
NEW GUINEA							
MN SPEAKERS	948	O. 936	10	1	1	0	
		E. 935.6	10.4	1.8	0.2		
NAN SPEAKERS	721	O. 521	101	63	36	1	1.364
		E. 524.9	97.5	57.4	41.2		

HAPLOTYPES

		1 5	1	1 2	REF.
MN SPEAKERS	F.	0.894	0.105	0.001	40
	S.E.	0.016	0.016	0.001	
NAN SPEAKERS	F.	0.561	0.368	0.071	40
	S.E.	0.017	0.016	0.007	

TABLE VI-2
TESTED FOR GM 1, 2, 3, 5, 6, 13, 14

PHENOTYPES

Population	Total		1 3 5 13 14	1	1 2 3 5 13 14	1 2	1 5 13 14	1 2 5 13 14	CHI SQ. DF	VALUE
MELANESIANS										
OCEANIA										
INDONESIA										
N. E. COAST W. NEW GUINEA	120	O.	112	7			1		0	
		E.	112.0	7.0			1.0			
S. W. COAST W. NEW GUINEA	262	O.	1	5		0	248	8	1	1.383
		E.	1.0	4.4		1.1	248.7	6.8		
PAP. N. GUINEA										
NEW GUINEA										
NORTH FORE NAN E. HIGHLANDS	113	O.	3	67	2	0	40	1	0	
		E.	3.0	66.7	2.3	0.0	40.3	0.6		
SOUTH FORE NAN E. HIGHLANDS	82	O.	7	48	3	2	21	1	1	3.312
		E.	8.6	46.6	4.7	0.3	20.8	0.9		
PAWAIAN NAN E. HIGHLANDS	29	O.	14	2			13		0	
		E.	14.0	2.0			13.0			
SIMBARI NAN E. HIGHLANDS	206	O.	24	48	18	3	105	8	2	1.741
		E.	24.9	49.7	16.0	2.0	102.2	11.1		
USURUFA NAN E. HIGHLANDS	98	O.	5	68	3	0	20	2	0	
		E.	4.9	66.8	4.2	0.1	21.3	0.6		
YAMBES SEPIK DIST.	37	O.	14	23					0	
		E.	14.0	23.0						
TENCH ISLAND	38	O.	30	4	3	1			1	0.198
		E.	30.3	3.8	2.6	1.4				
SOLOMON IS.										
BELLONA ISLAND	80	O.	55	7	12	6			1	0.126
		E.	55.5	6.6	11.3	6.6				
RENNELL ISLAND	62	O.	41	2	9	10			1	3.088
		E.	38.6	3.6	12.7	7.1				

HAPLOTYPES

Population		1 3 5 13 14	1	1 2	1 5 13 14	REF.
N. E. COAST W. NEW GUINEA	F.	0.742	0.242		0.017	168
	S.E.	0.044	0.044		0.016	
S. W. COAST W. NEW GUINEA	F.	0.002	0.130	0.015	0.853	168
	S.E.	0.002	0.030	0.005	0.030	
NORTH FORE NAN E. HIGHLANDS	F.	0.013	0.768	0.013	0.205	168
	S.E.	0.008	0.030	0.008	0.029	
SOUTH FORE NAN E. HIGHLANDS	F.	0.056	0.754	0.037	0.153	168
	S.E.	0.018	0.036	0.015	0.030	
PAWAIAN NAN E. HIGHLANDS	F.	0.281	0.263		0.457	168
	S.E.	0.065	0.090		0.096	
SIMBARI NAN E. HIGHLANDS	F.	0.068	0.491	0.073	0.368	168
	S.E.	0.013	0.029	0.013	0.028	
USURUFA NAN E. HIGHLANDS	F.	0.026	0.826	0.026	0.123	168
	S.E.	0.011	0.028	0.011	0.025	
YAMBES SEPIK DIST.	F.	0.212	0.788			168
	S.E.	0.051	0.051			
TENCH ISLAND	F.	0.632	0.314	0.054		168
	S.E.	0.075	0.073	0.026		
BELLONA ISLAND	F.	0.593	0.288	0.119		168
	S.E.	0.050	0.049	0.026		
RENNELL ISLAND	F.	0.585	0.241	0.175		168
	S.E.	0.056	0.054	0.036		

TABLE VI-2 CONTINUED
TESTED FOR GM 1, 2, 3, 5, 6, 13, 14

PHENOTYPES

MELANESIANS / OCEANIA / SOLOMON IS. / BOUGAINVILLE	TOTAL		1 3 5 13 14	1 3 5 13	1 2 3 5 13 14	1 2	CHI SQ. DF	CHI SQ. VALUE
ALL MN SPEAKERS	351	O.	329	2	20		1	2.036
		E.	330.0	1.3	18.2	1.5		
ALL NAN SPEAKERS	1813	O.	1668	44	93	8	1	5.865
		E.	1673.3	39.5	83.8	16.4		
ARAWA VILLAGE	MN 108	O.	101	1	6	0	0	
		E.	101.4	0.7	5.3	0.6		
ROROVANA VILLAGE	MN 243	O.	228	1	14	0	0	
		E.	228.6	0.6	12.9	0.9		
ATAMO VILLAGE	NAN 124	O.	117		6	1	0	
		E.	116.1		7.7	0.1		
BAIRIMA VILLAGE	NAN 59	O.	53		4	2	0	
		E.	51.3		7.5	0.3		
BOIRA VILLAGE	NAN 93	O.	93				0	
		E.						
KARNAVITU VILLAGE	NAN 133	O.	124	4	5	0	0	
		E.	124.5	3.5	4.1	0.9		
KOPANI VILLAGE	NAN 190	O.	187		2	1	0	
		E.	186.0		4.0	0.0		
KOPIKIRI VILLAGE	NAN 70	O.	66	1	3	0	0	
		E.	66.2	0.8	2.6	0.4		
KORPEI VILLAGE	NAN 181	O.	173	8			0	
		E.	173.0	8.0				

HAPLOTYPES

Population		1 3 5 13 14	1	1 2	REF.
ALL MN SPEAKERS	F.	0.910	0.062	0.028	33
	S.E.	0.025	0.024	0.006	
ALL NAN SPEAKERS	F.	0.824	0.148	0.028	33
	S.E.	0.011	0.011	0.003	
ARAWA VILLAGE	F.	0.890	0.082	0.028	33
	S.E.	0.046	0.045	0.011	
ROROVANA VILLAGE	F.	0.921	0.050	0.029	33
	S.E.	0.030	0.029	0.008	
ATAMO VILLAGE	F.	0.968		0.032	33
	S.E.	0.011		0.011	
BAIRIMA VILLAGE	F.	0.932		0.068	33
	S.E.	0.023		0.023	
BOIRA VILLAGE	F.	1.000			33
	S.E.				
KARNAVITU VILLAGE	F.	0.819	0.163	0.019	33
	S.E.	0.042	0.041	0.008	
KOPANI VILLAGE	F.	0.989		0.011	33
	S.E.	0.005		0.005	
KOPIKIRI VILLAGE	F.	0.871	0.108	0.021	33
	S.E.	0.058	0.057	0.012	
KORPEI VILLAGE	F.	0.790	0.210		33
	S.E.	0.036	0.036		

TABLE VI-2 CONTINUED
TESTED FOR GM 1, 2, 3, 5, 6, 13, 14

MELANESIANS
OCEANIA
SOLOMON IS.

PHENOTYPES

		TOTAL	1 3 5 13 14	1	1 2 3 5 13 14	1 2	DF	CHI SQ VALUE
BOUGAINVILLE								
MORONEI VILLAGE	NAN 112	O.	99		13	0	0	
		E.	99.4		12.2	0.4		
NASIWOIWA VILLAGE	NAN 128	O.	124	1	3	0	0	
		E.	124.2	0.9	2.7	0.3		
NUPATORO VILLAGE	NAN 99	O.	75	1	21	2	0	
		E.	76.0	0.6	19.2	3.3		
OKOWAPAIPA VILLAGE	NAN 94	O.	76	18			0	
		E.	76.0	18.0				
OLD SIUAI VILLAGE	NAN 26	O.	22	1	3	0	0	
		E.	22.4	0.7	2.3	0.6		
POMAUA VILLAGE	NAN 116	O.	110	4	2	0	0	
		E.	110.2	3.8	1.6	0.4		
RUMBA VILLAGE	NAN 148	O.	128	3	17	0	1	3.691
		E.	129.6	1.9	14.1	2.4		
SIERONJI VILLAGE	NAN 62	O.	62				0	
		E.						
TURUNGUM VILLAGE	NAN 88	O.	73		13	2	0	
		E.	71.8		15.4	0.8		
URUTO VILLAGE	NAN 90	O.	86	3	1	0	0	
		E.	86.1	2.9	0.8	0.2		
NASIOI RUMBA VILLAGE	NAN 161	O.	147	2	11	1	1	0.232
		E.	147.3	1.8	10.4	1.5		

HAPLOTYPES

	1 3 5 13 14	1	1 2	REF.
F.	0.942		0.058	33
S.E.	0.016		0.016	
F.	0.906	0.082	0.012	33
S.E.	0.043	0.043	0.007	
F.	0.803	0.076	0.121	33
S.E.	0.044	0.041	0.024	
F.	0.562	0.438		33
S.E.	0.046	0.046		
F.	0.779	0.164	0.058	33
S.E.	0.092	0.089	0.033	
F.	0.811	0.181	0.009	33
S.E.	0.045	0.045	0.006	
F.	0.830	0.112	0.057	33
S.E.	0.038	0.037	0.014	
F.	1.000			33
S.E.				
F.	0.903		0.097	33
S.E.	0.022		0.022	
F.	0.815	0.179	0.006	33
S.E.	0.052	0.051	0.006	
F.	0.858	0.104	0.038	167
S.E.	0.037	0.036	0.011	

81

TABLE VI-3
TESTED FOR GM 1, 2, 3, 5, 6, 13, 14, 21

PHENOTYPES

MELANESIANS OCEANIA SOLOMON IS.	TOTAL		P1 1·3·5·13·14	P2 1·3·5·13·14·21	P3 1·21	P4 1·2·3·5·13·14·21	P5 1·2·21	P6 1·5·13·14·21	P7 1·2·5·13·14·21	P8 1·5·13·14	P10 1·2·3·5·13·13·14	P11 1·2·5·13·14	DF	CHI SQ VALUE	REF.
BOUGAINVILLE															
AITA NAN	307	O.	50	127	76	30	24						2	3.378	167
		E.	53.8	126.0	73.8	23.5	30.0								
NAGOVISI NAN	386	O.	350	17	0	18	0	0			1	0	0		167
		E.	350.8	16.2	0.2	17.2	0.6	0.0			1.0	0.0			
NEW GUINEA															
HUI.I S. HIGHLANDS	149	O.			40	14		58	5	32			2	4.023	168
		E.			38.3	10.7		64.4	8.5	27.1					
ONABASULA S. HIGHLANDS	231	O.	0		3	32		91		105			2	8.558	168
		E.	2.0		1.0	27.0		102.9		98.1					
BAIMI W. DISTRICT	245	O.				17		77		151			1	2.606	168
		E.				12.6		85.9		146.6					
OLSOBIP W. DISTRICT	92	O.			33			33		26			1	7.132	168
		E.			26.6			45.7		19.6					
SOLOMON IS.															
MALAITA															
BAEGU MN	147	O.	92		50	3	0		2				1	1.627	167
		E.	93.1		46.1	5.7	1.6		0.4						
KWAIO MN	451	O.	399		36	1	13		2				1	1.225	167
		E.	397.7		37.3	0.9	14.4		0.8						
LAU MN	143	O.	78		41	4	11	0	3		6	0	3	3.696	167
		E.	80.1		38.5	4.6	8.6	2.3	2.0		6.7	0.1			

HAPLOTYPES

MELANESIANS
OCEANIA
SOLOMON IS.

			1 3 5 14	1 3 21	1 2 21	1 5 13 14	1 2 5 13 14	REF.
	TOTAL							
BOUGAINVILLE								
AITA NAN	307	F.	0.419	0.490	0.091			167
		S.E.	0.020	0.020	0.012			
NAGOVISI NAN	386	F.	0.953	0.022	0.023		0.001	167
		S.E.	0.008	0.005	0.005		0.001	
NEW GUINEA								
HULI S. HIGHLANDS	149	F.	0.507	0.067		0.426		168
		S.E.	0.029	0.015		0.029		
ONABASULA S. HIGHLANDS	231	F.	0.006	0.342		0.652		168
		S.E.	0.004	0.022		0.022		
BAIMI W. DISTRICT	245	F.	0.227			0.773		168
		S.E.	0.019			0.019		
OLSOBIP W. DISTRICT	92	F.	0.538			0.462		168
		S.E.	0.037			0.037		
SOLOMON IS.								
MALAITA								
BAEGU MN	147	F.	0.796	0.197	0.007			167
		S.E.	0.024	0.023	0.005			
KWAIO MN	451	F.	0.939	0.044	0.017			167
		S.E.	0.008	0.007	0.004			
LAU MN	143	F.	0.748	0.180	0.040		0.031	167
		S.E.	0.026	0.023	0.012		0.010	

83

TABLE VI-4
TESTED FOR GM 1, 2, 3, 5, 6, 11, 13, 16, 21, 24

PHENOTYPES

		1 3 5 11 13 13	1 3 5 11 13 21	1 21	1 2 3 5 11 13 21	1 2 21	1 5 11 13 21	1 2 5 11 13 21	1 5 11 13	CHI SQ. DF	CHI SQ. VALUE	REF.
MELANESIANS												
OCEANIA												
FIJI	TOTAL											
LAU ISLANDS	O.	10	35	13	13	3				2	10.272	139
74	E.	15.6	29.2	13.7	7.5	7.9						
VITI LEVU	O.	19	70	108	23	46	4	1	0	2	3.674	139
271	E.	17.0	79.0	101.3	17.8	50.8	4.2	0.9	0.0			
PAP. N. GUINEA												
NEW BRITAIN												
KILENGE	O.	59	15	0						0		139
74	E.	59.8	13.5	0.8								
NEW GUINEA												
ALL. MN SPEAKERS	O.	239	67	1			75		155	2	15.608	139
537	E.	253.6	48.8	9.7			75.9		149.0			
ALL. NAN SPEAKERS	O.	2	12	50	2	30	161	27	257	3	42.814	139
541	E.	10.5	4.4	41.6	0.9	18.9	195.3	40.2	229.0			
ASMAT NAN AGATS VILLAGE	O.				3	3	35	9	129	2	1.300	139
179	E.				2.7	1.7	36.8	10.4	127.4			
AWIN NAN FLY RIVER	O.				3	0	62	3	65	2	7.276	139
133	E.				8.7	0.8	49.8	2.2	71.5			
YANGGAN NAN FLY RIVER	O.				1	1	28	2	59	1	1.353	139
91	E.				2.6	0.5	25.2	2.5	60.2			
WAFFA NAN MARKHAM VALL.	O.	2	12	43	2	26	36	13	4	4	4.610	139
138	E.	3.9	9.2	44.5	2.6	28.7	33.4	9.4	6.3			

HAPLOTYPES

MELANESIANS							
OCEANIA							
FIJI	TOTAL		1 3 5 11 13	1 21	1 2 21	1 5 11 13	REF.
LAU ISLANDS	74	F.	0.459	0.430	0.110		139
		S.E.	0.041	0.041	0.027		
VITI LEVU	271	F.	0.238	0.611	0.138	0.013	139
		S.E.	0.018	0.021	0.015	0.005	
PAP. N. GUINEA							
NEW BRITAIN							
KILENGE	74	F.	0.899	0.101			139
		S.E.	0.025	0.025			
NEW GUINEA							
ALL MN SPEAKERS	537	F.	0.339	0.134		0.527	139
		S.E.	0.016	0.010		0.017	
ALL NAN SPEAKERS	541	F.	0.015	0.277	0.057	0.651	139
		S.E.	0.004	0.014	0.007	0.014	
ASMAT NAN AGATS VILLAGE	179	F.		0.122	0.035	0.844	139
		S.E.		0.017	0.010	0.019	
AWIN NAN FLY RIVER	133	F.		0.256	0.011	0.733	139
		S.E.		0.027	0.006	0.027	
YANGGAN NAN FLY RIVER	91	F.		0.170	0.017	0.813	139
		S.E.		0.028	0.010	0.029	
WAFFA NAN MARKHAM VALL.	138	F.	0.059	0.568	0.160	0.213	139
		S.E.	0.014	0.031	0.023	0.025	

85

TABLE VI-4 CONTINUED
TESTED FOR GM 1,2,3,5,6,11,13,16,21,24

PHENOTYPES

MELANESIANS

OCEANIA

PAP. N. GUINEA

		TOTAL	1 3 5 11 13	1 3 5 11 13 21	1 2 3 5 11 13 21	1 5 11 13 21	1 2 5 11 13	DF	CHI SQ. VALUE	REF.
NEW GUINEA										
AWAN VILLAGE	MN 102	O.	50	15	0	12	25	2	4.108	139
		E.	53.5	10.5	1.8	12.9	23.3			
INTOAP VILLAGE	MN 84	O.	50	2	0	6	26	1	1.019	139
		E.	49.1	3.1	0.2	4.5	27.1			
ITSINGATS VILLAGE	MN 66	O.	21	14	0	17	14	2	6.896	139
		E.	24.6	9.4	3.6	14.3	14.0			
PUGUAP VILLAGE	MN 90	O.	35	6	1	12	36	2	0.171	139
		E.	35.7	5.2	1.1	12.6	35.5			
SINGAS VILLAGE	MN 87	O.	35	9	0	13	30	2	2.536	139
		E.	37.1	6.5	1.4	12.8	29.3			
YANUF VILLAGE	MN 41	O.	22	6	0	2	11	1	2.618	139
		E.	24.0	3.4	0.4	3.8	9.4			
YATSING VILLAGE	MN 67	O.	26	15	0	13	13	2	5.797	139
		E.	29.7	10.2	2.9	12.0	12.2			

HAPLOTYPES

			1 3 5 11 13	1 21	1 2 21	1 5 11 13	REF.
MELANESIANS							
OCEANIA							
PAP. N. GUINEA	TOTAL						
NEW GUINEA							
AWAN VILLAGE	MN 102	F. S.E.	0.390 0.039	0.132 0.024		0.478 0.040	139
INTOAP VILLAGE	MN 84	F. S.E.	0.385 0.043	0.048 0.016		0.567 0.044	139
ITSINGATS VILLAGE	MN 66	F. S.E.	0.305 0.044	0.235 0.037		0.460 0.047	139
PUGUAP VILLAGE	MN 90	F. S.E.	0.261 0.035	0.111 0.023		0.628 0.039	139
SINGAS VILLAGE	MN 87	F. S.E.	0.293 0.038	0.126 0.025		0.580 0.040	139
YANUF VILLAGE	MN 41	F. S.E.	0.424 0.063	0.098 0.033		0.479 0.064	139
YATSING VILLAGE	MN 67	F. S.E.	0.364 0.047	0.209 0.035		0.427 0.048	139

TABLE VI-5
TESTED FOR GM 1, 2, 3, 5, 6, 11, 13, 15, 16, 17, 21

PHENOTYPES

			1 17 21	1 2 17 21	1 5 13 17 21	1 2 5 11 13 17 21	1 5 11 13 17	CHI SQ.	
								DF	VALUE
MELANESIANS									
OCEANIA									
PAP. N. GUINEA	TOTAL								
NEW GUINEA									
ENGA LAIAGAM VILL.	NAN 185	O. E.	114 114.4	23 21.3	41 41.7	2 3.7	5 3.8	2	1.319

HAPLOTYPES

	1 17 21	1 2 17 21	1 5 11 13 17	REF.
F.	0.787	0.070	0.143	18
S.E.	0.021	0.014	0.018	

TABLE VI-6
TESTED FOR GM 1, 2, 3, 5, 6, 10, 11, 13, 14, 15, 16, 17, 21, 23, 24

PHENOTYPES

MELANESIANS
OCEANIA
PAP. N. GUINEA

NEW BRITAIN
TOLAI MN

Location	TOTAL	O/E	1 3 5 10 11 13 14 23	1 3 50 11 13 14 17 23 14	1 3 5 10 11 13 14 17 21 23	1 3 5 10 11 13 14 17 21	1 17 17 21	1 2 3 50 10 11 14 17 21	1 2 3 50 11 14 17 21 23	1 3 50 10 11 14 17 23	1 3 50 11 13 14 17 21 23	1 5 10 11 13 14 17 21 23	1 2 50 10 11 14 17 21 23	1 5 10 11 14 17 23	DF	CHI SQ. VALUE	REF.
BUNAMIN VILLAGE	55	O.	7	0	5	1	8	23	2	9					3	18.343	19
		E.	9.1	0.1	10.1	1.0	3.4	14.0	1.4	15.8							
OMITTING GM(2)	55	O.	7	0	28	3	17								1	1.451	
		E.	9.1	0.1	24.1	2.5	19.2										
KOULON VILLAGE	45	O.	19	0	8	1	4	6	1	5	1	0	0	0	2	2.903	19
		E.	16.6	0.2	11.4	1.3	2.4	7.2	0.8	4.0	0.6	0.2	0.1	0.0			
KURAIP VILLAGE	39	O.	12	0	2	0	2	13	2	8					2	2.191	19
		E.	10.7	0.1	4.3	0.5	0.5	13.1	1.5	8.2							
RAKUNAI VILLAGE	17	O.	1		6		2	1		7					2	2.803	19
		E.	1.2		4.1		3.5	2.6		5.7							
RALMALMAL VILLAGE	68	O.	23	3	19	4	3	8	4	2	2	0	0	0	4	4.681	19
		E.	26.9	2.2	14.5	5.5	3.4	6.8	2.6	4.0	1.3	0.5	0.2	0.0			
VAIRIKI VILLAGE	56	O.	20	0	7	3	0	13	4	9					3	2.932	19
		E.	19.2	0.9	6.8	1.8	0.9	14.5	3.8	8.1							
VUNALAKA VILLAGE	18	O.	3	2	1	0	4	6	0	2					3	11.971	19
		E.	3.6	0.4	3.3	1.6	1.5	2.8	1.3	3.5							
OMITTING GM(2)	18	O.	3	2	7	0	6								1	0.938	
		E.	3.6	0.4	6.1	2.9	5.0										
VUNALIA VILLAGE	48	O.	10	0	9	2	1	12	3	8	2	0	0	1	5	2.511	19
		E.	11.6	0.4	7.3	1.5	1.6	10.9	2.3	8.5	2.0	0.7	1.1	0.1			

HAPLOTYPES

MELANESIANS

OCEANIA

PAP. N. GUINEA

NEW BRITAIN

TOLAI   MN

Population	TOTAL		1·3·5·10·11·13·14·23	1·3·5·10·11·13·14	1·5·10·11·13·14·17	1·7·21	1·2·17·21	1·5·10·11·13·14·17·23	REF.
BUNAMIN VILLAGE	55	F.	0.371	0.038	0.248		0.342		19
		S.E.	0.048	0.022	0.046		0.050		
' OMITTING GM(2)	55	F.	0.371	0.038	0.591		0.047		
		S.E.	0.048	0.022					
KOULON VILLAGE	45	F.	0.549	0.063	0.231		0.147	0.011	19
		S.E.	0.058	0.036	0.046		0.039	0.011	
KURAIP VILLAGE	39	F.	0.471	0.055	0.118		0.357		19
		S.E.	0.061	0.034	0.042		0.058		
RAKUNAI VILLAGE	17	F.	0.265		0.451		0.285		19
		S.E.	0.076		0.092		0.084		
RALMALMAL VILLAGE	68	F.	0.474	0.180	0.225		0.106	0.015	19
		S.E.	0.049	0.041	0.036		0.027	0.010	
VAIRIKI VILLAGE	56	F.	0.475	0.124	0.128		0.274		19
		S.E.	0.053	0.039	0.035		0.044		
VUNALAKA VILLAGE	18	F.	0.321	0.152	0.289		0.238		19
		S.E.	0.083	0.067	0.080		0.076		
' OMITTING GM(2)	18	F.	0.321	0.152	0.528				
		S.E.	0.083	0.067	0.083				
VUNALIA VILLAGE	48	F.	0.414	0.086	0.183		0.275	0.042	19
		S.E.	0.055	0.036	0.043		0.049	0.020	

89

TABLE VI-6 CONTINUED
TESTED FOR GM 1, 2, 3, 5, 6, 10, 11, 13, 14, 15, 16, 17, 21, 23, 24

PHENOTYPES

MELANESIANS
OCEANIA
PAP. N. GUINEA

		Gm 1 3 5 10 11 13 14 23	Gm 1 3 5 10 11 13 14 17 23	Gm 1 3 5 10 11 13 14 17 21	Gm 1 17 21	Gm 1 2 3 5 10 11 13 14 17 21 23	Gm 1 2 3 5 10 11 13 14 17 21	Gm 1 2 17 21	Gm 1 3 5 10 11 13 14 17 23	Gm 1 3 5 10 11 13 14 17 21	Gm 1 5 10 11 13 14 17 21	Gm 1 2 5 10 11 13 14 17	Gm 1 5 10 11 13 14 17	CHI SQ. DF	VALUE	REF.
TOTAL																
NEW BRITAIN																
BAINING NAN 43 GAULIM VILLAGE	O.	3	5		4	7		24						2	1.107	19
	E.	1.9	5.5		4.1	8.7		22.8								
SULKA NAN 54 MOPE VILLAGE	O.	20	9	4	1	8	2	4	4	1	0	0	0	5	2.707	19
	E.	21.4	8.8	2.8	1.5	7.5	2.4	3.6	2.5	0.8	0.8	0.7	0.1			
TOLAI MN 40 NORDUP VILLAGE	O.	17	1	0	0	12	3	3	0	1	0	0	0	1	1.763	19
	E.	18.2	0.7	0.3	0.0	10.0	4.7	3.0	0.5	0.2	0.0	0.3	0.0			

HAPLOTYPES

MELANESIANS
OCEANIA
PAP. N. GUINEA

		Gm 1 3 5 10 11 13 14 23	Gm 1 3 5 10 11 13 14 17 23	Gm 1 3 5 10 11 13 14 17 21	Gm 1 2 17 21	Gm 1 5 10 11 13 14 17	REF.
TOTAL							
NEW BRITAIN							
BAINING NAN 43 GAULIM VILLAGE	F.	0.209	0.307	0.483			19
	S.E.	0.044	0.060	0.064			
SULKA NAN 54 MOPE VILLAGE	F.	0.493	0.165	0.155	0.141	0.046	19
	S.E.	0.055	0.037	0.044	0.034	0.020	
TOLAI MN 40 NORDUP VILLAGE	F.	0.484	0.228	0.258	0.017	0.050 0.013	19
	S.E.	0.065	0.058	0.050	0.016	0.013 0.012	

91

PHENOTYPES

MELANESIANS
OCEANIA
PAP. N. GUINEA

GM phenotype patterns (column headers, read vertically):

1 3 5 10 11 13 14 17 21
1 2 3 5 10 11 13 14 17 21
1 3 5 10 11 13 14 17 21 23
1 3 5 10 11 13 14 17 23
1 2 5 10 11 13 14 17 21 23
1 5 10 11 13 14 17 23
1 3 5 10 11 13 14 17
1 5 10 11 13 14 17 21
1 2 5 10 11 13 14 17 21
1 5 10 11 13 14 17

Population		Observed / Expected values	CHI SQ DF	VALUE	REF.
TOTAL					
NEW GUINEA					
GOGODARA NAN 99	O.	2 12 80 2 3	1	1.135	19
BALIMO VILLAGE	E.	0.8 13.4 79.2 2.9 2.7			
KUMAN NAN 101	O.	0 0 13 51 1 25 3 1 1 5 0 1	3	5.739	19
MINJ VILLAGE	E.	0.0 1.4 12.6 51.5 0.3 21.9 2.5 3.6 0.1 6.0 0.7 0.2			

HAPLOTYPES

MELANESIANS
OCEANIA
PAP. N. GUINEA

GM haplotype patterns (column headers, read vertically):

1 3 5 10 11 13 14 17 21 23
1 5 10 11 13 14 17 23
1 5 10 11 13 14 17

Population		Frequency / S.E. values	REF.
TOTAL			
NEW GUINEA			
GOGODARA NAN 99	F.	0.091 0.745 0.164	19
BALIMO VILLAGE	S.E.	0.020 0.046 0.043	
KUMAN NAN 101	F.	0.010 0.714 0.083 0.152 0.041	19
MINJ VILLAGE	S.E.	0.007 0.032 0.020 0.026 0.015	

TABLE VI-6 CONTINUED
TESTED FOR GM 1, 2, 3, 5, 6, 10, 11, 13, 14, 15, 16, 17, 21, 23, 24

PHENOTYPES

MELANESIANS

OCEANIA

PAP. N. GUINEA

1	1	1		1	1	1
3	3	3		3	3	5
5	5	5	1	5	5	10
10	10	10	3	10	10	11
11	11	11	10	11	11	13
13	13	13	11	13	13	14
14	14	14	13	14	14	17
23		21	14	17	17	23
		23	17	23	21	
			21		23	

TOTAL

NEW GUINEA

		CHI SQ.	
		DF VALUE	REF.

MOTU   MN 38 O. 23   7   0   0   6   0   1
POREBADA VILL.   E. 22.3 7.3 0.4 0.0 7.1 0.1 0.4   0   0.4   19

HAPLOTYPES

MELANESIANS

OCEANIA

PAP. N. GUINEA

1	1		1
3	3		5
5	5	1	10
10	10	3	11
11	11	10	13
13	13	11	14
14	14	17	17
23	21	21	23

TOTAL

REF.

NEW GUINEA

MOTU   MN 38 F.   0.444 0.437 0.013 0.105
POREBADA VILL.   S.E. 0.072 0.072 0.013 0.035   19

TABLE VII-1
TESTED FOR GM 1, 2, 5, 6

PHENOTYPES

MICRONESIANS

OCEANIA

		1	1		CHI SQ.
MARSHALL IS.	TOTAL	5	1	DF	VALUE
RONGELAP	149	O. 146	3	3.0	0
ATOLL		E. 146.0			0

HAPLOTYPES

	1	1	REF.
	5	1	
F.	0.858	0.142	162
S.E.	0.041	0.041	

TABLE VII-2
TESTED FOR GM 1, 2, 3, 5, 6, 13, 14, 21

PHENOTYPES

MICRONESIANS OCEANIA CAROLINE IS.	TOTAL		1 3 5 13 14	1 3 5 13 14 21	1 3 14 21	1 2 5 13 14 21	1 3 6 13 14	1 3 6 21	1 2 5 6 21	1 5 6	1 5 13 14 21	1 2 5 13 14 21	1 5 6 13 14	1 5 13 14	CHI SQ. DF	CHI SQ. VALUE	REF.
KUSAIEANS	254	O.	200	34	3	0	4	0	0	0					2	3.218	172
		E.	200.2	35.5	1.6	1.2	3.6	0.3	0.1	0.0							
MOKILESE	207	O.	117	55	12	6	12	3	0	0					3	10.630	172
		E.	110.9	64.2	9.3	1.8	11.0	3.2	0.3	0.3							
PINGELAPESE	409	O.	354	38	1	3	6	1	0	0					2	9.556	172
		E.	351.2	40.5	1.2	0.5	6.5	0.4	0.1	0.0							
PONAPEANS	190	O.	105	67	9	4	1	0	0		2	0	0	0	2	0.598	172
		E.	106.1	64.8	10.4	4.4	0.7	0.2	0.0		1.7	0.1	0.0	0.1			

HAPLOTYPES

MICRONESIANS OCEANIA CAROLINE IS.	TOTAL		1 3 5 13 14	1 3 14 21	1 2 21	1 5 6	1 5 13 14	REF.
KUSAIEANS	254	F.	0.888	0.079	0.026		0.008	172
		S.E.	0.014	0.012	0.007		0.004	
MOKILESE	207	F.	0.732	0.212	0.020		0.036	172
		S.E.	0.022	0.020	0.007		0.009	
PINGELAPESE	409	F.	0.927	0.053	0.011		0.009	172
		S.E.	0.009	0.008	0.004		0.003	
PONAPEANS	190	F.	0.728	0.234	0.016	0.003	0.019	172
		S.E.	0.025	0.022	0.006	0.003	0.013	

TABLE VII-3
TESTED FOR GM 1, 2, 3, 5, 6, 11, 13, 16, 21, 24

MICRONESIANS

OCEANIA

CAROLINE IS.

PHENOTYPES

	TOTAL		1,3,5,11,13	1,3,5,11,13,21	1,2,3,5,11,13,21	1,2,21	2,21	DF	CHI SQ. VALUE
WEST TRUK	48	O.	20	15	2	6	5	2	1.103
		E.	19.4	14.6	2.7	7.6	3.6		

HAPLOTYPES

	1,3,5,11,13	1,21	2,21	REF.
F.	0.635	0.239	0.125	139
S.E.	0.049	0.044	0.035	

TABLE VIII-1
TESTED FOR GM 1, 2, 3

MONGOLOIDS

ASIA

VIETNAM

PHENOTYPES

	TOTAL		1	1,2	1,3	1,2,3	DF	CHI SQ. VALUE
VIETNAMESE	414	O.	6	7	361	40	1	0.008
		E.	5.9	7.2	361.1	39.8		

HAPLOTYPES

	1	1,2	1,3	REF.
F.	0.119	0.058	0.822	185
S.E.	0.022	0.008	0.023	

TABLE VIII-2
TESTED FOR GM 1,2,5

PHENOTYPES

		TOTAL	1	1 2	1 5	1 2 5	5	DF	CHI SQ. VALUE
MONGOLOIDS									
ASIA									
INDIA									
THARUS KUMAON REGION	O.	152	7	7	106	32		1	2.360
	E.		5.3	10.4	108.6	27.7			
MIYAKO									
RYUKYU ISLANDERS	O.	200	62	58	53	27		1	2.604
	E.		58.0	62.8	57.9	21.3			
OKINAWA									
RYUKYU ISLANDERS	O.	200	85	62	44	9		1	0.698
	E.		86.9	59.9	41.9	11.3			
MACAO									
CHINESE	O.	499	16	7	432	41	3	1	1.042
	E.		14.6	9.6	433.7	38.1	3.0		
REP OF CHINA									
CHINESE NORTH	O.	161	28	22	92	19		1	0.033
	E.		28.3	21.5	91.6	19.6			
CHINESE SOUTH	O.	143	5	7	112	19		1	0.056
	E.		5.2	6.6	111.7	19.5			
TAIWAN									
ABORIGINES									
AMI	O.	225	1	0	221	3		0	
	E.		0.9	0.2	221.1	2.8			
ATAYAL	O.	263	7	0	252	4		0	
	E.		6.6	0.7	252.4	3.3			

HAPLOTYPES

		1	1 2	1 5	5	REF.
THARUS KUMAON REGION	F.	0.187	0.134	0.679		17
	S.E.	0.035	0.020	0.037		
RYUKYU ISLANDERS (MIYAKO)	F.	0.538	0.239	0.223		90
	S.E.	0.027	0.023	0.022		
RYUKYU ISLANDERS (OKINAWA)	F.	0.659	0.198	0.143		90
	S.E.	0.025	0.021	0.018		
CHINESE (MACAO)	F.	0.171	0.049	0.702	0.078	123
	S.E.	0.021	0.007	0.030	0.022	
CHINESE NORTH	F.	0.420	0.137	0.444		90
	S.E.	0.033	0.020	0.032		
CHINESE SOUTH	F.	0.191	0.096	0.713		90
	S.E.	0.037	0.018	0.039		
AMI	F.	0.063	0.007	0.930		90
	S.E.	0.032	0.004	0.033		
ATAYAL	F.	0.159	0.008	0.834		90
	S.E.	0.030	0.004	0.030		

TABLE VIII-2 CONTINUED TESTED FOR GM 1,2,5

PHENOTYPES

		TOTAL	1	1 2	1 5	1 2 5	5	CHI SQ. DF	VALUE
MONGOLOIDS									
ASIA									
TAIWAN									
ABORIGINES									
BUNUN	O.	103	1	0	95	7		0	
	E.		0.7	0.7	95.4	6.2			
PAIWAN	O.	178	7	9	137	25		1	0.001
	E.		7.0	8.9	136.9	25.1			
CHINESE	O.	200	9	7	169	15		1	0.498
	E.		9.8	5.7	168.1	16.5			
S. AMERICA									
BOLIVIA									
AYMARA INDIANS *	O.	1459	1241	112	100	6		1	0.579
	E.		1239.5	113.5	101.5	4.5			
CHIPAYA INDIANS	O.	96	96					0	
	E.								
MOCETENES INDIANS	O.	76	20	55	1	0		0	
	E.		20.4	54.6	0.5	0.5			
PECHEURS INDIANS	O.	311	269	36	6	0		0	
	E.		269.3	35.7	5.6	0.4			
QUECHUA INDIANS	O.	131	86	20	20	4	1	1	1.077
	E.		84.7	21.4	21.3	2.5	1.1		

HAPLOTYPES

		1	1 2	1 5	5	REF.
BUNUN	F.	0.081	0.034	0.885		90
	S.E.	0.045	0.013	0.046		
PAIWAN	F.	0.199	0.101	0.701		90
	S.E.	0.033	0.016	0.034		
CHINESE	F.	0.221	0.057	0.722		90
	S.E.	0.032	0.012	0.033		
AYMARA INDIANS *	F.	0.922	0.041	0.037		105
	S.E.	0.005	0.004	0.004		
CHIPAYA INDIANS	F.	1.000				105
	S.E.					
MOCETENES INDIANS	F.	0.518	0.476	0.007		136
	S.E.	0.049	0.049	0.007		
PECHEURS INDIANS	F.	0.931	0.060	0.010		105
	S.E.	0.010	0.010	0.004		
QUECHUA INDIANS	F.	0.804	0.096	0.010	0.090	136
	S.E.	0.025	0.019	0.044	0.043	

* EXCLUDING SEVEN GM(5) SAMPLES.

TABLE VIII-2 CONTINUED
TESTED FOR GM 1,2,5

PHENOTYPES

	TOTAL		1	1;2	1;5	1;2;5	5	CHI SQ. DF	VALUE
MONGOLOIDS									
S. AMERICA									
FRENCH GUIANA									
EMERILLON INDIANS	40	O.	25	15				0	
		E.	25.0	15.0					
GALIBI INDIANS	191	O.	78	88	15	10		1	1.002
		E.	76.2	89.9	17.1	7.7			
OAYANA INDIANS	97	O.	60	36	1	0		0	
		E.	60.2	35.8	0.8	0.2			
OYAMPI INDIANS	98	O.	65	33				0	
		E.	65.0	33.0					
PALIKOAR INDIANS	75	O.	15	56	1	3		1	0.732
		E.	14.4	56.6	1.8	2.2			
VENEZUELA									
PARAUJANO INDIANS	114	O.	19	14	48	22	11	1	2.640
		E.	16.4	17.9	50.7	17.4	11.6		

HAPLOTYPES

		1	1;2	1;5	5		REF.
EMERILLON INDIANS	F.	0.791	0.209				28
	S.E.	0.048	0.048				
GALIBI INDIANS	F.	0.632	0.301	0.067			28
	S.E.	0.027	0.026	0.013			
OAYANA INDIANS	F.	0.788	0.207	0.005			28
	S.E.	0.031	0.031	0.005			
OYAMPI INDIANS	F.	0.814	0.186				28
	S.E.	0.029	0.029				
PALIKOAR INDIANS	F.	0.438	0.535	0.027			28
	S.E.	0.051	0.051	0.013			
PARAUJANO INDIANS	F.	0.379	0.169	0.133	0.319	0.044	28
	S.E.	0.039	0.026	0.051	0.044		

99

TABLE VIII-3
TESTED FOR GM 1, 2, 13

PHENOTYPES

MONGOLOIDS			1	1 2	1 13	13	DF	CHI SQ. VALUE
C. AMERICA								
MEXICO	TOTAL							
CHIPAS INDIANS AGUACATENANGO	156	O.	77	74	3	2		
		E.	76.5	74.5	3.6	1.4	1	0.129

HAPLOTYPES

	1	1 2	1 13	REF.
F.	0.700	0.284	0.016	26
S.E.	0.028	0.028	0.007	

TABLE VIII-4
TESTED FOR GM 1, 2, 3, 5

PHENOTYPES

MONGOLOIDS			1	1 2	1 3 5	1 2 3 5	1 5	1 2 5	3 5	DF	CHI SQ. VALUE
ASIA											
KOREA	TOTAL										
KOREANS *	114	O.	47	34	25	7			1		
		E.	47.1	33.9	24.9	7.2			1.0	0	0
KOREANS	107	O.	53	30	18	4	1	1			
		E.	52.6	30.4	17.8	4.2	1.6	0.4		1	0.017
VIETNAM											
VIETNAMESE	232	O.	6	2	201	20	1	1	1		
		E.	4.8	3.9	202.0	18.3	1.5	0.5	1.0	1	1.736

HAPLOTYPES

	1	1 2	1 3 5	1 5	3 5	REF.
F.	0.643	0.200	0.064		0.093	5
S.E.	0.034	0.028	0.049		0.046	
F.	0.701	0.179	0.109		0.011	46
S.E.	0.033	0.028	0.022		0.007	
F.	0.144	0.050	0.719	0.020	0.066	45
S.E.	0.030	0.010	0.045	0.014	0.033	

* EXCLUDING ONE GM(1,3) SAMPLE.

TABLE VIII-5
TESTED FOR GM 1, 2, 3, 6

PHENOTYPES

MONGOLOIDS

S. AMERICA

L. TITICACA

BOLIVIA	TOTAL		1	1 2	1 3	1 2 3	CHI SQ. DF	VALUE
AMANTANI INDIANS	54	O.	50	3	1	0	0	
		E.	50.0	3.0	1.0	0.0		
AYMARA INDIANS *	1845	O.	1526	182	119	18	1	14.861
		E.	1516.3	191.9	129.0	7.8		
GUAQUI INDIANS	90	O.	76	12	2	0	0	
		E.	76.1	11.9	1.9	0.1		
LLACHON INDIANS	54	O.	48	6			0	
		E.	48.0	6.0				
PUNO INDIANS	74	O.	60	11	3	0	0	
		E.	60.2	10.8	2.8	0.2		
TAQUILE INDIANS	39	O.	35	4			0	
		E.	35.0	4.0				

HAPLOTYPES

		1	1 2	1 3	REF.
AMANTANI INDIANS	F.	0.963	0.028	0.009	15
	S.E.	0.018	0.016	0.009	
AYMARA INDIANS *	F.	0.907	0.056	0.038	15
	S.E.	0.005	0.004	0.003	
GUAQUI INDIANS	F.	0.920	0.069	0.011	15
	S.E.	0.021	0.019	0.008	
LLACHON INDIANS	F.	0.943	0.057		15
	S.E.	0.023	0.023		
PUNO INDIANS	F.	0.902	0.077	0.020	15
	S.E.	0.025	0.022	0.012	
TAQUILE INDIANS	F.	0.947	0.053		15
	S.E.	0.026	0.026		

* EXCLUDING TEN GM(3) SAMPLES.

101

TABLE VII-6
TESTED FOR GM 1, 2, 5, 6

MONGOLOIDS
ASIA

PHENOTYPES

	TOTAL		1	1 2	1 5	1 5 6	1 2 5	1 2 5 6	5	CHI SQ. DF	CHI SQ. VALUE
JAPAN											
KAWASAKA-SHI	258	O.	135	74	40		9			1	0.002
		E.	135.1	73.9	39.9		9.1				
KUMAMOTO	516	O.	276	144	77		19			1	0.193
		E.	274.7	145.4	78.5		17.4				
OSAKA	748	O.	346	261	101		40			1	1.833
		E.	340.7	266.7	107.1		33.5				
TOKYO	109	O.	53	35	18		3			1	0.545
		E.	54.1	33.8	16.8		4.3				
MALAYSIA											
CHINESE KUALA LUMPUR	90	O.	4	2	81		3			1	0.743
		E.	4.5	1.2	80.5		3.8				
CHINESE KUALA LUMPUR	149	O.	7	4	122		14		2	1	0.094
		E.	6.7	4.5	122.3		13.4		2.0		
INDIANS-TAMILS AND SIKHS	60	O.	16	11	26		6		1	0	
		E.	16.0	10.9	25.9		6.1		1.0		
MALAYS-PERLIS	156	O.	4	3	132		16		1	1	0.164
		E.	3.7	3.6	132.4		15.3		1.0		
THAILAND											
BANGKOK	163	O.	8	6	132		17			1	0.005
		E.	7.9	6.1	132.1		16.8				

HAPLOTYPES

		1	1 2	1 5	1 5 6	5	REF.
KAWASAKA-SHI	F.	0.724	0.176	0.100			1
	S.E.	0.021	0.018	0.014			
KUMAMOTO	F.	0.730	0.173	0.098			183
	S.E.	0.014	0.012	0.009			
OSAKA	F.	0.675	0.226	0.099			157
	S.E.	0.013	0.012	0.008			
TOKYO	F.	0.704	0.194	0.102			115
	S.E.	0.033	0.028	0.021			
CHINESE KUALA LUMPUR	F.	0.223	0.028	0.749			152
	S.E.	0.050	0.012	0.050			
CHINESE KUALA LUMPUR	F.	0.212	0.062	0.610		0.116	188
	S.E.	0.037	0.014	0.055		0.041	
INDIANS-TAMILS AND SIKHS	F.	0.517	0.154	0.200		0.129	188
	S.E.	0.051	0.034	0.075		0.064	
MALAYS-PERLIS	F.	0.154	0.063	0.704		0.080	188
	S.E.	0.036	0.014	0.054		0.040	
BANGKOK	F.	0.221	0.073	0.706			188
	S.E.	0.035	0.015	0.036			

TABLE VIII-6, CONTINUED
TESTED FOR GM 1,2,5,6

PHENOTYPES

	TOTAL		1	1 2	1 5	1 2 5	1 5 6	1 2 5 6	5	CHI SQ. DF	CHI SQ. VALUE
MONGOLOIDS											
N. AMERICA											
U.S.A.											
ATHABASCAN IND. ARCTIC VILL. AL.	58	O.	34	24						0	
		E.	34.0	24.0							
ATHABASCAN IND. FORT YUKON AL.	51	O.	33	16	2	0				0	
		E.	33.3	15.7	1.7	0.3					
ESKIMOS WAINWRIGHT AL.	50	O.	38	2	9	1				0	
		E.	37.4	2.7	9.6	0.3					
OCEANIA											
U.S.A.											
FILIPINOS HONOLULU, HI.	138	O.	1	1	115	11			10	0	
		E.	0.9	1.3	115.2	10.7			10.0		
S. AMERICA											
BRAZIL											
AWEIKOMA IND. SANTA CATARINA	58	O.	28	29	1	0				0	
		E.	28.2	28.7	0.7	0.3					
CAINGANG IND. SANTA CATARINA	52	O.	26	23	3	0				0	
		E.	26.7	22.3	2.2	0.8					
CAINGANG MEST. SANTA CATARINA	107	O.	40	23	32	9	0	1	2	0	
		E.	38.8	24.5	32.6	8.1	0.8	0.2	2.0		
*	104	O.	40	23	32	9				1	0.356
		E.	39.0	24.2	33.2	7.7					
GUARINI IND. SANTA CATARINA	34	O.	18	13	3	0				1	0.224
		E.	18.6	12.4	2.4	0.7					

HAPLOTYPES

Population		1	1 2	1 5	1 5 6	5	REF.
ATHABASCAN IND. ARCTIC VILL. AL.	F.	0.766	0.234				153
	S.E.	0.042	0.042				
ATHABASCAN IND. FORT YUKON AL.	F.	0.808	0.172	0.020			153
	S.E.	0.041	0.039	0.014			
ESKIMOS WAINWRIGHT AL.	F.	0.864	0.030	0.105			153
	S.E.	0.035	0.017	0.032			
FILIPINOS HONOLULU, HI.	F.	0.080	0.044	0.606	0.269		124
	S.E.	0.038	0.012	0.056	0.041		
AWEIKOMA IND. SANTA CATARINA	F.	0.698	0.293	0.009			137
	S.E.	0.047	0.046	0.009			
CAINGANG IND. SANTA CATARINA	F.	0.716	0.255	0.029			137
	S.E.	0.048	0.046	0.017			
CAINGANG MEST. SANTA CATARINA	F.	0.602	0.167	0.088	0.005	0.138	137
	S.E.	0.036	0.027	0.052	0.005	0.048	
*	F.	0.612	0.167	0.221			
	S.E.	0.036	0.027	0.031			
GUARINI IND. SANTA CATARINA	F.	0.739	0.216	0.045			137
	S.E.	0.056	0.053	0.026			

* EXCLUDING TWO GM(5) AND ONE GM(1,2,5,6) SAMPLES.

TABLE VIII-6 CONTINUED
TESTED FOR GM 1,2,5,6

MONGOLOIDS

S. AMERICA

		PHENOTYPES								CHI SQ.		HAPLOTYPES					REF.
BRAZIL	TOTAL		1	1 2	1 5	1 2 5	1 5 6	1 2 5 6	5	DF	VALUE	1	1 2	1 5	1 5 6	5	
XAVANTE IND. MATO GROSSO	73	O.	51	22							0	F. 0.836	0.164				91
		E.	51.0	22.0								S.E. 0.032	0.032				
PARAGUAY																	
NORTHWEST																	
AYORE INDIANS	71	O.	70	1							0	F. 0.993	0.007				14
		E.	70.0	1.0								S.E. 0.007	0.007				
CHEROTI INDIANS	28	O.	24	4							0	F. 0.926	0.074				14
		E.	24.0	4.0								S.E. 0.036	0.036				
CHULUPI INDIANS	121	O.	85	36							0	F. 0.838	0.162				14
		E.	85.0	36.0								S.E. 0.025	0.025				
GUARAYU INDIANS	14	O.	13	1							0	F. 0.964	0.036				14
		E.	13.0	1.0								S.E. 0.036	0.036				
LENGUA INDIANS	45	O.	41	4							0	F. 0.955	0.045				14
		E.	41.0	4.0								S.E. 0.022	0.022				
SANAPANA INDIANS	97	O.	69	28							0	F. 0.843	0.157				14
		E.	69.0	28.0								S.E. 0.027	0.027				
TAPIETE INDIANS	19	O.	19								0	F. 1.000					14
		E.										S.E.					
TOBA INDIANS	42	O.	34	8							0	F. 0.900	0.100				14
		E.	34.0	8.0								S.E. 0.034	0.034				
SOUTHWEST																	
GUAYAKI INDIANS	61	O.	29	32							0	F. 0.689	0.311				14
		E.	29.0	32.0								S.E. 0.046	0.046				

104

TABLE VIII-7
TESTED FOR GM 1, 2, 3, 5, 6

PHENOTYPES

MONGOLOIDS
C. AMERICA
MEXICO

	TOTAL		1	1 2	1 3 5	1 2 3 5	1 5 6	1 2 5	1 5 6	1 2 5 6	1 3 5 6	3 5	DF	CHI SQ. VALUE	REF.
CUAJINICUILPA	63	O.	25	4	15	0	11	1	4	2	1	0			
		E.	25.1	4.7	12.2	0.9	11.3	0.9	5.6	0.4	0.9	1.0	3	4.817	164
		E.	24.4	4.7	14.1	1.0	11.0	0.9	5.6	0.4		1.0	2	3.220	
OMETEPEC	82	O.	33	15	13	6	8	2	2	0	0	3			
		E.	30.7	16.9	17.1	3.8	7.8	1.8	1.4	0.3	0.3	1.9	3	3.383	164
POCHUTLA	89	O.	31	11	23	6	12	2	2	0	0	2			
		E.	30.5	12.8	22.8	3.7	12.0	2.1	1.4	0.2	0.4	3.1	3	2.065	164
SAN PEDRO MIXTEPEC	94	O.	43	12	17	3	13	1	2	0	0	3			
		E.	42.3	12.0	19.8	2.3	12.2	1.5	1.5	0.2	0.3	1.8	3	2.081	164

HAPLOTYPES

MONGOLOIDS
C. AMERICA
MEXICO

	TOTAL		1	1 2	1 3 5	1 2 3 5	1 5 6	1 5 6	3 5	REF.
CUAJINICUILPA	63	F.	0.631	0.057		0.129	0.057		0.127	
		S.E.	0.046	0.021		0.034	0.021		0.030	
		F.	0.622	0.057	0.137	0.127		0.057		164
		S.E.	0.047	0.021	0.032	0.034		0.021		
OMETEPEC	82	F.	0.611	0.150	0.074	0.012	0.152			164
		S.E.	0.040	0.029	0.023	0.009	0.028			
POCHUTLA	89	F.	0.585	0.112	0.106	0.011	0.185			164
		S.E.	0.040	0.024	0.027	0.008	0.029			
SAN PEDRO MIXTEPEC	94	F.	0.671	0.089	0.091	0.011	0.138			164
		S.E.	0.036	0.021	0.023	0.008	0.025			

TABLE VIII-8
TESTED FOR GM 1, 2, 3, 5, 10

PHENOTYPES

	TOTAL	1	1;2	1;3;5;10	1;2;3;5;10	DF	CHI SQ. VALUE	REF.
MONGOLOIDS								
ASIA								
NORTH VIETNAM								
VIETNAMESE KINH * — O.	149	1	2	125	21	0	0	54
E.		0.8	2.6	125.5	20.1			
N. AMERICA								
CANADA								
LABRADOR INDIANS — O.	47	21		8	17	1	0.5	128
E.		20.7		8.9	16.8			

HAPLOTYPES

	1	1;2	1;3;5;10	3;5;10
VIETNAMESE KINH * — F.	0.071	0.080	0.849	
S.E.	0.035	0.016	0.037	
LABRADOR INDIANS — F.	0.664		0.229	0.106
S.E.	0.054		0.049	0.032

* EXCLUDING TWO GM(1,2,3) AND TWO GM(1,3,10) SAMPLES.

TABLE VIII-9
TESTED FOR GM 1, 2, 3, 5, 10, 11

PHENOTYPES

MONGOLOIDS
ASIA
BHUTAN

		1	1 2 3 5 10 11	1 3 5 10 11	1 2 3 5 10 11	1 2 10 11	1 5 10 11	1 2 5 10 11	DF	CHI SQ. VALUE	REF.

BHUTANI *

	TOTAL	1	1 2	1 3 5 10 11	1 2 3 5 10 11	1 2 10 11	1 5 10 11	1 2 5 10 11	DF	CHI SQ. VALUE	REF.
O.	150	36	37	38	9	23	5	2	0			
E.		38.4	34.1	37.3	9.8	21.3	7.1	1.5	0.5	2	1.217	89

HAPLOTYPES

MONGOLOIDS
ASIA
BHUTAN

	TOTAL	1	1 2	1 3 5 10 11	1 10 11	1 5 10 11	REF.
F.	150	0.506	0.189	0.172	0.125	0.008	
S.E.		0.032	0.024	0.023	0.022	0.006	89

* EXCLUDING ONE GM(1, 3, 5) SAMPLE.

TABLE VIII-10
TESTED FOR GM 1, 2, 3, 5, 13, 15

PHENOTYPES

MONGOLOIDS	TOTAL		1	1 2	1 3 5 13	1 2 3 5 13	1 3 5 13 15	1 2 3 5 13 15	1 3 5 13 15	1 3 5 13	DF	CHI SQ. VALUE	REF.
ASIA													
JAPAN													
JAPANESE	98	O.	28	15	15	3	26	7	4		3	0.687	75
		E.	27.9	16.1	13.9	3.2	26.4	5.6	5.0				
N. AMERICA													
GREENLAND													
ESKIMOS SOUTHWEST	212	O.	109	8	45	1	34	1	11	3	4	3.164	94
		E.	107.8	7.3	44.9	1.5	37.4	1.2	7.2	4.7			
ESKIMOS WEST	75	O.	36	1	14	0	20	0	3	1	0		75
		E.	36.5	0.7	13.7	0.1	19.6	0.2	3.2	1.0			

HAPLOTYPES

MONGOLOIDS	TOTAL		1	1 2	1 3 5 13	1 3 5 13 15	3 5 13	REF.
ASIA								
JAPAN								
JAPANESE	98	F.	0.533	0.136	0.120	0.211		75
		S.E.	0.038	0.025	0.024	0.031		
N. AMERICA								
GREENLAND								
ESKIMOS SOUTHWEST	212	F.	0.713	0.024	0.114	0.149		94
		S.E.	0.022	0.007	0.016	0.017		
ESKIMOS WEST	75	F.	0.697	0.007	0.014	0.168	0.114	75
		S.E.	0.039	0.007	0.007	0.058	0.032 0.057	

TABLE VIII-11
TESTED FOR GM 1, 2, 5, 13, 16, 21

PHENOTYPES

MONGOLOIDS

ASIA

JAPAN

	TOTAL	1;21	1 2;21	1 13 16;21	1 2 13 16;21	1 13 16;21	1 5 13;21	1 2 5 13;21	1 5 13 16	1 5 13	CHI SQ. DF	CHI SQ. VALUE	REF.
JAPANESE	287	O. 77	45	71	19	10	37	9	13	6	5	2.762	184
		E. 79.4	46.4	64.7	16.7	13.2	37.3	9.7	15.2	4.4			

HAPLOTYPES

MONGOLOIDS

ASIA

JAPAN

	TOTAL	1 21	1 2 21	1 13 16	1 5 13	REF.
JAPANESE	287	F. 0.526	0.136	0.214	0.124	184
		S.E. 0.021	0.015	0.017	0.014	

TABLE VIII-12
TESTED FOR GM 1, 2, 3, 5, 6, 13, 14

PHENOTYPES

MONGOLOIDS	TOTAL		1	1 2	1 3 5 13 14	1 2 3 5 13 14	1 13 14	1 2 13	1 5 13 14	1 2 5 13 14	1 3 5 13 14	DF	CHI SQ. VALUE	REF.
ASIA														
JAPAN														
JAPANESE	166	O.	33	32	29	6	55	11				2	1.315	158
		E.	35.3	29.1	29.0	6.0	52.3	14.3						
REP OF CHINA														
CHINESE	100	O.	11	8	49	16	12	4				2	2.984	158
		E.	9.3	11.2	52.2	11.8	11.1	4.3						
TAIWAN														
CHINESE	100	O.		0	87	7	4	2				1	0.009	158
		E.		0.2	87.1	6.8	4.1	1.8						
THAILAND														
THAIS	479	O.	7	7	416	40	4	1			4	2	0.160	160
		E.	7.0	7.2	416.4	39.4	3.6	1.4			4.0			
THAIS	228	O.	4	2	190	31	1	0				0		161
		E.	2.8	5.0	192.3	26.9	0.6	0.4						
C. AMERICA														
MEXICO														
CHOLS INDIANS *	139	O.	66	46	12	1	9	3	1	1		2	1.451	164
		E.	66.6	45.2	10.3	2.7	9.4	2.7	1.6	0.4				
CORAS INDIANS	98	O.	53	16	7	2	20	0				1	0.850	164
		E.	54.0	15.0	8.1	0.9	17.9	2.2						

* EXCLUDING THREE GM(3,5,13,14) SAMPLES.

HAPLOTYPES

	TOTAL		1	1 2	1 3 5 13 14	1 13	1 3 13 14	1 5 13 14	3 5 13 14	REF.
MONGOLOIDS										
ASIA										
JAPAN										
JAPANESE	166	F.	0.461	0.162	0.112	0.265				158
		S.E.	0.032	0.021	0.018	0.028				
REP OF CHINA										
CHINESE	100	F.	0.305	0.148	0.400	0.147				158
		S.E.	0.042	0.026	0.040	0.034				
TAIWAN										
CHINESE	100	F.		0.045	0.753	0.202				158
		S.E.		0.015	0.047	0.046				
THAILAND										
THAIS	479	F.	0.121	0.051	0.708	0.028			0.091	160
		S.E.	0.021	0.007	0.031	0.012			0.023	
THAIS	228	F.	0.111	0.073	0.804	0.011				161
		S.E.	0.029	0.012	0.031	0.011				
C. AMERICA										
MEXICO										
CHOLS INDIANS	139	F.	0.692	0.205	0.048	0.047	0.008			164
		S.E.	0.029	0.026	0.013	0.013	0.005			
CORAS INDIANS	98	F.	0.742	0.097	0.047	0.114	0.024			164
		S.E.	0.033	0.022	0.015	0.024				

TABLE VIII-12 CONTINUED
TESTED FOR GM 1,2,3,5,6,13,14

PHENOTYPES

MONGOLOIDS	TOTAL		1	1 2	1 3 5 13 14	1 2 3 5 13 14	1 3 13	1 2 13	1 5 13 14	1 2 5 13 14	CHI SQ. DF	VALUE	REF.
C. AMERICA													
MEXICO													
HAUSTECOS INDIANS	173	O.	92	53	2	2	16	6	2	0	2	1.886	164
		E.	90.0	55.1	3.2	0.8	17.4	4.5	1.6	0.4			
MAZATECOS INDIANS	122	O.	74	31	6	2	4	1	4	0	2	0.842	164
		E.	73.7	31.3	6.8	1.2	4.2	0.8	3.4	0.6			
ZAPATECOS INDIANS *	95	O.	72	9	11	1	1	0	1	0	0		164
		E.	71.8	9.2	11.3	0.7	0.9	0.1	0.9	0.1			
N. AMERICA													
U.S.A.													
ATHABASCAN INDIANS, ALASKA	64	O.	26	17	3	0	12	6			1	1.494	158
		E.	24.8	18.3	2.4	0.6	14.0	3.9					
S. AMERICA													
BRAZIL.													
XAVANTE IND.													
SAO DOMINGOS	73	O.	51	22							0		150
		E.	51.0	22.0									
SAO MARCOS	248	O.	152	96							0		150
		E.	152.0	96.0									
SIMOES LOPES	143	O.	85	58							0		150
		E.	85.0	58.0									

* EXCLUDING THREE GM(3,5,13,14) SAMPLES.

HAPLOTYPES

MONGOLOIDS	TOTAL		1	1 2	1 3 5 14	1 3 13	1 5 13 14	3 5 13 14	REF.
C. AMERICA									
MEXICO									
HAUSTECOS INDIANS	173	F.	0.721	0.194	0.012	0.067	0.006		164
		S.E.	0.025	0.023	0.006	0.014	0.004		
MAZATECOS INDIANS	122	F.	0.777	0.151	0.033	0.022	0.017		164
		S.E.	0.028	0.024	0.012	0.010	0.008		
ZAPATECOS INDIANS	95	F.	0.869	0.054	0.065	0.006	0.006	0.006	164
		S.E.	0.025	0.017	0.018	0.006	0.006	0.006	
N. AMERICA									
U. S. A.									
ATHABASCAN INDIANS, ALASKA	64	F.	0.623	0.198	0.024	0.156			158
		S.E.	0.046	0.037	0.014	0.034			
S. AMERICA									
BRAZIL									
XAVANTE IND.									
SAO DOMINGOS	73	F.	0.836	0.164					150
		S.E.	0.032	0.032					
SAO MARCOS	248	F.	0.783	0.217					150
		S.E.	0.020	0.020					
SIMOES LOPES	143	F.	0.771	0.229					150
		S.E.	0.027	0.027					

TABLE VIII-13
TESTED FOR GM 1, 2, 3, 5, 10, 11, 21

PHENOTYPES

			1 2 1 ;21	1 2 ;21	1 3 5 10 11 ;21	1 2 3 5 10 11 ;21	1 3 5 10 11 ;21	1 5 10 11 ;21	1 2 10 11 ;21	1 10 11	3 5 10 11	CHI SQ. DF	VALUE	REF.
MONGOLOIDS														
N. AMERICA														
GREENLAND	TOTAL													
ESKIMOS	55	O.	27	2	4	1	0	19	0	2	0	2	1.026	98
JULIANEHAB		E.	28.3	2.2	3.6	0.1	1.0	16.5	0.6	2.4	0.1	2	1.026	
		E.	28.3	2.2	3.6	0.1	1.2	16.5	0.6	2.4				

HAPLOTYPES

			1 ;21	1 2 ;21	1 3 5 10 11	1 5 10 11	3 5 10 11	REF.
MONGOLOIDS								
N. AMERICA								
GREENLAND	TOTAL							
ESKIMOS	55	F.	0.718	0.028	0.209	0.045		98
JULIANEHAB		S. E.	0.043	0.016	0.039	0.020		
		F.	0.718	0.028	0.045	0.209	0.039	
		S. E.	0.043	0.016	0.020	0.039		

TABLE VIII-14
TESTED FOR GM 1, 2, 3, 5, 11, 13, 15

PHENOTYPES

MONGOLOIDS
N. AMERICA
GREENLAND

	TOTAL		1	1 2	1 3 5 11 13	1 2 3 5 11 13	1 3 11 13 15	1 2 11 13 15	1 3 5 11 13 15	3 5 11 13	DF	CHI SQ. VALUE	REF.
ESKIMOS ANGMAGSSALIK	283	O.	183		2	97	1				0		94
		E.	182.6		2.4	97.4	0.6						
ESKIMOS THULE	150	O.	116			34					0		94
		E.	116.0			34.0							
MIXED THULE	95	O.	46	2	9	37	0	0	1		1	3.074	94
		E.	48.0	1.4	7.8	34.5	0.1	2.4	0.3				

HAPLOTYPES

MONGOLOIDS
N. AMERICA
GREENLAND

	TOTAL		1	1 2	1 3 5 11 13	1 3 11 13 15	3 5 13	REF.
ESKIMOS ANGMAGSSALIK	283	F.	0.803		0.005	0.191		94
		S.E.	0.018		0.003	0.017		
ESKIMOS THULE	150	F.	0.879		0.121			94
		S.E.	0.019		0.019			
MIXED THULE	95	F.	0.711	0.011	0.221	0.058		94
		S.E.	0.035	0.007	0.032	0.017		

TABLE VIII-15
TESTED FOR GM 1, 2, 3, 5, 6, 13, 14, 21

PHENOTYPES

		TOTAL	1 21	1 2 21	1 3 5 13 14 21	1 2 3 5 13 14 21	1 3 5 13 14	1 3 13 21	1 2 13 21	1 13	1 5 6 21	1 3 5 6 13 14	1 5 6	3 5 13 14	CHI SQ. DF	VALUE	REF.
MONGOLOIDS																	
ASIA																	
JAPAN																	
JAPANESE	O.	87	17	23	9	4	4	17	7	6							165
	E.		17.7	21.6	8.0	3.9	4.9	17.7	8.7	4.4					4	1.321	
MALAYSIA																	
ABORIGINES	O.	68	0	0	5	4	59										169
	E.		0.1	0.2	4.7	3.7	59.3								0		
SEMAI	O.	175	0		2		171				0	2	0				169
	E.		0.0		2.0		171.0				0.0	2.0	0.0		0		
N. AMERICA																	
CANADA																	
ESKIMOS IGLOOLIK	O.	365	227	4	22	0	6	91	0	14				1			85
	E.		223.3	3.2	23.5	0.2	5.1	97.8	0.7	10.7				0.6	3	2.162	
GREENLAND																	
ESKIMOS AUGPILAGTOK IS. UPERNAVIK DIST.	O.	144	63	4	47	1	6	12	0	0				11			174
	E.		62.0	3.4	49.9	1.3	4.7	11.8	0.3	0.6				10.0	3	1.393	

116

HAPLOTYPES

			21	1 2 21	1 3 5 13 14	1 13	1 5 6	3 5 13 14	REF.
MONGOLOIDS									
ASIA									
JAPAN	TOTAL								
JAPANESE	87	F.	0.451	0.221	0.102	0.226			165
		S.E.	0.039	0.033	0.023	0.032			
MALAYSIA									
ABORIGINES	68	F.	0.037	0.029	0.934				169
		S.E.	0.016	0.015	0.021				
SEMAI	175	F.	0.006		0.989		0.006		169
		S.E.	0.004		0.006		0.004		
N. AMERICA									
CANADA									
ESKIMOS IGLOOLIK	365	F.	0.782	0.005		0.171		0.041	85
		S.E.	0.015	0.003		0.014		0.007	
GREENLAND									
ESKIMOS AUGPILAGTOK IS. UPERNAVIK DIST.	144	F.	0.656	0.018		0.062		0.264	174
		S.E.	0.028	0.008		0.014		0.026	

TABLE VIII-15 CONTINUED
TESTED FOR GM 1, 2, 3, 5, 6, 13, 14, 21

PHENOTYPES

MONGOLOIDS S. AMERICA BRAZIL	TOTAL	1 3 5 13 21 / 1 2 21	1 2 13 21 / 1 3 5 13 14 21	1 3 5 13 14 21 / 1 3 5 13 14 21	1 2 13 21 / 1 3 13 21	1 5 6 21 / 1 5 6 13 14	1 3 5 6 13 14	1 5 6	3 5 13 14	CHI SQ. DF VALUE	REF.
CAYAPO IND.											
KUBEN-KRAN-KEGN *	132	O. 100 32	E. 100.0 32.0							0	138
MEKRANOTI #	90	O. 48 42	E. 48.0 42.0							0	138
TXUKAHAMAE	154	O. 78 75	E. 77.4 75.6	0 0.7	1 0.3	0 0.0				0	138
XIKRIN	59	O. 47 12	E. 47.0 12.0							0	138

* EXCLUDING TWO GM(1,5,13,14,21) SAMPLES.

EXCLUDING ONE GM(1,3,5,13,14,21) AND ONE GM(1,2,3,5,13,14,21) SAMPLES.

HAPLOTYPES

MONGOLOIDS S. AMERICA BRAZIL	TOTAL	1 3 5 13 14 / 1 2 21	1 2 13	1 3 5 6 13 14	REF.
CAYAPO IND.					
KUBEN-KRAN-KEGN	132	F. 0.870 0.130	S.E. 0.021 0.021		138
MEKRANOTI	90	F. 0.730 0.270	S.E. 0.036 0.036		138
TXUKAHAMAE	154	F. 0.709 0.288	S.E. 0.028 0.028	0.003 0.003	138
XIKRIN	59	F. 0.893 0.107	S.E. 0.029 0.029		138

TABLE VIII-16.
TESTED FOR GM 1, 2, 3, 5, 10, 14, 17, 21 *

PHENOTYPES

MONGOLOIDS
N. AMERICA
GREENLAND

	TOTAL		1 17 21	1 2 17 21	3 5 10 14 17 21	1 2 3 5 10 14 17 21	1 10 17 21	1 2 10 17 21	1 3 5 10 14 17	1 10 17	3 5 10 14	DF	CHI SQ. VALUE	REF.
ESKIMOS ANGMAGSSALIK #	40	O.	34	1	2	1					2	2	0.3	98
		E.	31.5	1.8	6.2	0.2					0.3			
ESKIMOS WEST COAST @	45	O.	15	1	12	1	6	0	7	0	3	3	4.033	98
		E.	13.3	1.1	14.1	0.6	7.1	0.3	3.8	0.9	3.8			
POLAR ESKIMOS THULE	27	O.	24				3			0		0		98
		E.	24.1				2.8			0.1				

HAPLOTYPES

MONGOLOIDS
N. AMERICA
GREENLAND

	TOTAL		1 17 21	1 2 17 21	1 10 17	3 5 10 14	REF.
ESKIMOS ANGMAGSSALIK	40	F.	0.887	0.025	0.087		98
		S.E.	0.035	0.018	0.032		
ESKIMOS WEST COAST	45	F.	0.544	0.022	0.144	0.289	98
		S.E.	0.053	0.016	0.037	0.049	
POLAR ESKIMOS THULE	27	F.	0.944		0.056		98
		S.E.	0.031		0.031		

* OMITTING GM(11).

EXCLUDING ONE GM(1,5,10,17,21) SAMPLE.

@ EXCLUDING ONE GM(1,2,3,17,21), ONE GM(1,3,14,17,21), ONE GM(1,3,5,10,17,21), AND ONE GM(1,5,10,17,21) SAMPLES.

TABLE VIII-17
TESTED FOR GM 1, 2, 3, 5, 13, 15, 16, 21

PHENOTYPES

MONGOLOIDS

ASIA

INDONESIA	TOTAL		21	1 2 21	1 3 5 13 21	1 2 3 5 13 21	1 3 5 13	1 13 15 16 21	1 2 13 15 16 21	1 3 5 13 15 16	1 13 15 16	CHI SQ. DF	VALUE	REF.
INDONESIANS JAVA	183	O.	2	7	37	34	101	0	0	2	0	2	0.696	82
		E.	2.9	8.0	34.4	32.5	103.3	0.3	0.2	1.5	0.0			
JAPAN														
JAPANESE OSAKA	236	O.	49	36	23	10	4	62	23	16	13	5	2.640	77
		E.	48.4	39.5	25.8	9.0	3.4	57.5	20.0	15.3	17.1			
JAPANESE OSAKA	343	O.	72	54	37	13	7	82	34	25	19	5	2.974	78
		E.	69.5	57.8	40.1	14.2	5.8	80.6	28.5	23.2	23.4			
TAIWAN														
CHINESE TAICHUNG CITY	286	O.	15	12	83	29	120	8	3	16	0	4	0.712	83
		E.	15.1	12.3	84.4	29.5	118.4	6.2	2.2	17.4	0.6			
ABORIGINES														
ATAYAL	154	O.	1	2	44	5	102					2	3.256	79
		E.	3.7	1.2	39.3	5.9	103.9							
BUNUN	104	O.	7	1	32	6	58					2	1.194	79
		E.	5.3	1.7	34.7	5.2	57.0							
PAIWAN	210	O.	7	7	67	17	110	0	0	2	0	2	0.950	79
		E.	9.0	5.9	63.5	18.1	111.5	0.4	0.1	1.5	0.0			

HAPLOTYPES

MONGOLOIDS

ASIA

	TOTAL		2 1	1 2 1	1 3 5 1 3	1 3 5 1 6	REF.
INDONESIA							
INDONESIANS JAVA	183	F.	0.125	0.118	0.751	0.005	82
		S.E.	0.018	0.017	0.023	0.004	
JAPAN							
JAPANESE OSAKA	236	F.	0.453	0.157	0.121	0.269	77
		S.E.	0.023	0.017	0.015	0.020	
JAPANESE OSAKA	343	F.	0.450	0.159	0.130	0.261	78
		S.E.	0.019	0.015	0.013	0.017	
TAIWAN							
CHINESE TAICHUNG CITY	286	F.	0.229	0.080	0.643	0.047	83
		S.E.	0.018	0.012	0.020	0.009	
ABORIGINES							
ATAYAL	154	F.	0.155	0.023	0.821		79
		S.E.	0.021	0.009	0.022		
BUNUN	104	F.	0.226	0.034	0.740		79
		S.E.	0.029	0.013	0.030		
PAIWAN	210	F.	0.207	0.059	0.729	0.005	79
		S.E.	0.020	0.012	0.022	0.003	

TABLE VIII-18
TESTED FOR GM 1, 2, 3, 5, 6, 11, 13, 16, 21 *

PHENOTYPES

MONGOLOIDS		TOTAL	1 21	1 2 21	1 3 5 11 13 21	1 2 3 5 11 13 21	1 3 5 11 13 21	1 11 13 16 21	1 2 11 13 16 21	1 3 5 11 13 16	1 11 13 16	DF	CHI SQ. VALUE	REF.
ASIA														
JAPAN														
MIE PREFECTURE #	O.	562	140	133	37	19	4	120	47	16	46	5	9.246	144
	E.		133.4	129.6	39.0	15.8	2.8	134.0	54.2	19.6	33.6			
NIIGATA PREFECTURE #	O.	193	36	35	15	6	3	50	22	11	15	5	1.253	144
	E.		35.7	35.9	16.3	6.8	1.9	48.6	20.2	11.1	16.5			
YAMAGATA PREFECTURE #	O.	195	39	21	14	3	2	68	17	10	21	5	1.808	144
	E.		41.0	22.2	14.2	3.4	1.2	62.8	15.2	10.9	24.1			
OKINAWA														
RYUKYUANS HANADA CITY @	O.	198	51	37	11	7	2	46	12	7	25	5	11.498	144
	E.		46.0	34.2	14.0	4.5	1.1	55.4	17.7	8.4	16.7			

* ACCORDING TO THE AUTHORS, "ALL SERA WERE TYPED FOR EITHER GM(11) OR GM(13)."

THE AUTHORS OMITTED THREE GM(1,16,21), TWO GM(1,2,16,21), ONE GM(1,2,16,21), ONE GM(1,5,11,13,16,21), ONE GM(1,2,3,5,11,13,16,21), ONE GM(1,5,11,13,16), ONE GM(1,5,11,13,21), ONE GM(1,2,11,13,16), AND ONE GM(1,16) SAMPLES, BUT DID NOT STATE FROM WHICH OF THESE POPULATIONS.

@ EXCLUDING ONE GM(1,2,5,11,13,21) AND ONE GM(1,5,11,13,16,21) SAMPLES.

HAPLOTYPES

MONGOLOIDS

ASIA

JAPAN

	TOTAL		21	121	135113	111316	REF.
MIE PREFECTURE	562	F.	0.487	0.197	0.071	0.245	144
		S.E.	0.015	0.013	0.008	0.013	
NIIGATA PREFECTURE	193	F.	0.430	0.179	0.098	0.293	144
		S.E.	0.026	0.020	0.015	0.023	
YAMAGATA PREFECTURE	195	F.	0.458	0.111	0.079	0.351	144
		S.E.	0.026	0.016	0.014	0.024	
OKINAWA							
RYUKYUANS HANADA CITY	198	F.	0.487	0.154	0.073	0.290	144
		S.E.	0.026	0.019	0.013	0.023	

TABLE VIII-19
TESTED FOR GM 1, 2, 3, 5, 6, 11, 16, 21, 24

PHENOTYPES

MONGOLOIDS	TOTAL		21 / 21	1 2 / 21	1 3 5 11 / 21	1 2 3 5 11 / 21	1 3 5 11 16 / 21	1 2 11 16 21 / 21	1 3 5 11 16 / 11 16	1 1 16 / 11 16	3 5 11 / 11	DF	CHI SQ. VALUE	REF.
ASIA														
HONG KONG														
CHINESE	203	O.	4	1	37	130	14	2	0	15	0	3	1.846	141
		E.	2.8	2.1	38.4	130.9	12.2	2.0	0.6	13.7	0.4			
N. AMERICA														
CANADA														
OJIBWA IND. PINKANGIKUM	102	O.	77	11			11	3		0		1	1.997	179
		E.	75.5	12.9			12.0	1.0		0.5				
OJIBWA IND. WIKWEMIKONG	117	O.	59	13	33	5	2	1	1	0	3	3	1.943	179
		E.	58.4	14.8	31.8	3.8	2.8	0.3	0.8	0.0	4.3			

HAPLOTYPES

MONGOLOIDS	TOTAL		21	1 2 / 21	1 3 5 11 16	1 3 5 11	REF.
ASIA							
HONG KONG							
CHINESE	203	F.	0.118	0.037	0.803	0.042	141
		S.E.	0.016	0.009	0.020	0.010	
N. AMERICA							
CANADA							
OJIBWA IND. PINKANGIKUM	102	F.	0.861	0.071	0.069		179
		S.E.	0.025	0.018	0.018		
OJIBWA IND. WIKWEMIKONG	117	F.	0.706	0.084	0.017	0.192	179
		S.E.	0.030	0.019	0.008	0.026	

TABLE VIII-20
TESTED FOR GM 1, 2, 3, 5, 6, 13, 16, 21, 24

PHENOTYPES

MONGOLOIDS — ASIA — KOREA

	TOTAL	21 / 21	1 2 / 21 21	1 3 5 13 / 21	1 2 3 5 13 / 21	1 3 5 13 / 21	1 3 13 16 / 21	1 2 13 16 / 21	1 3 5 13 / 16	1 13 / 16	CHI SQ. DF	CHI SQ. VALUE	REF.
KOREANS *	195												
O.		51	47	31	16	1	26	12	6	5	5	5.231	143
E.		50.2	51.1	27.9	11.7	3.9	27.4	11.5	7.6	3.7			

HAPLOTYPES

MONGOLOIDS — ASIA — KOREA

	TOTAL	21 / 21	1 2 / 21 21	1 3 5 13 / 21	1 3 13 / 16	REF.
KOREANS	195					143
F.		0.507	0.213	0.141	0.138	
S.E.		0.026	0.022	0.018	0.017	

* EXCLUDING FOUR GM(1,3,5,13,16,21), THREE GM(1,2,3,5,13,16,21), THREE GM(1,2,5,13,16,21), TWO GM(1,2,5,13,21), TWO GM(1,5,13,21), ONE GM(1,5,13,16,21), AND ONE GM(1,5,13) SAMPLES.

TABLE VIII-21
TESTED FOR GM 1, 2, 3, 5, 6, 11, 13, 16, 21, 24

PHENOTYPES

MONGOLOIDS
ASIA
REP OF CHINA

		TOTAL	21	1 2 21	1 3 5 11 13 21	1 3 5 11 13 21	1 2 3 5 11 13 21	1 3 11 16 21	1 2 11 13 16 21	1 3 5 11 13 16	1 11 13 16	CHI SQ. DF	VALUE	REF.
CHINESE NORTH *	O.	167	31	19	25	45	19	12	4	11	1	5	4.882	142
	E.		27.3	24.5	18.2	48.1	21.2	11.7	4.4	10.3	1.3			
CHINESE SOUTH *	O.	325	10	5	30	69	179	6	3	22	1	4	2.638	142
	E.		7.6	7.1	28.6	73.1	176.5	5.0	2.0	24.3	0.8			
TAIWAN ABORIGINES #														
AMI	O.	151	0	1	2	10	137	0	0	1	0	0		139
	E.		0.2	0.1	3.0	10.3	136.4	0.0	0.0	1.0	0.0			
ATAYAL	O.	126	3	1	7	39	75	0	0	1	0	1	0.867	139
	E.		4.2	1.6	6.3	35.9	77.0	0.2	0.0	0.8	0.0			
BUNUN	O.	36	1			9	26					0		139
	E.		0.8			9.3	25.8							
PAIWAN	O.	48	1	4	6	9	28					1	1.814	139
	E.		1.0	2.3	8.2	10.2	26.3							
OTHER TRIBES	O.	31	1	0	2	6	22					0		139
	E.		0.5	0.3	1.7	6.7	21.8							
CHINESE *	O.	208	9	10	24	60	87	5	0	12	1	4	0.916	142
	E.		10.0	9.4	23.1	59.3	87.6	4.2	1.6	12.3	0.4			

* THREE GM(1,3,5,11,13,16,21), THREE GM(1,5,11,13,21), ONE GM(1,2,5,11,13,21), ONE GM(1,2,5,11,13,21), ONE GM(1,2,3,13,16,21), ONE GM(1,2W,3,5,11,13,16), ONE GM(1,2W,3,5,11,13), ONE GM(1,3,13,16), AND ONE GM(1,2) SAMPLES WERE OMITTED, BUT THE AUTHOR DID NOT STATE FROM WHICH POPULATIONS. 2W=2 WEAK. WEAK WAS NOT DEFINED.

THE AUTHOR OMITTED ONE GM(1,3,5,13,16,21), ONE GM(1,3,21), AND ONE GM(1,3) SAMPLES, BUT DID NOT STATE FROM WHICH TRIBES.

MONGOLOIDS

ASIA

REP OF CHINA

	TOTAL		2 1	1 2 1	1 3 5 1 1 3	1 3 1 6	REF.
CHINESE NORTH	167	F.	0.404	0.153	0.356	0.087	142
		S.E.	0.027	0.020	0.026	0.015	
CHINESE SOUTH	325	F.	0.153	0.060	0.737	0.051	142
		S.E.	0.014	0.009	0.017	0.009	
TAIWAN							
ABORIGINES							
AMI	151	F.	0.036	0.010	0.950	0.003	139
		S.E.	0.011	0.006	0.013	0.003	
ATAYAL	126	F.	0.182	0.032	0.782	0.004	139
		S.E.	0.024	0.011	0.026	0.004	
BUNUN	36	F.	0.153		0.847		139
		S.E.	0.042		0.042		
PAIWAN	48	F.	0.144	0.116	0.740		139
		S.E.	0.037	0.034	0.045		
OTHER TRIBES	31	F.	0.129	0.032	0.839		139
		S.E.	0.043	0.023	0.047		
CHINESE	208	F.	0.220	0.086	0.649	0.046	142
		S.E.	0.020	0.014	0.023	0.010	

TABLE VIII-21 CONTINUED
TESTED FOR GM 1, 2, 3, 5, 6, 11, 13, 16, 21, 24

PHENOTYPES

MONGOLOIDS
ASIA
THAILAND

	TOTAL		21	1 2 21	1 3 5 11 13 21	1 2 3 5 11 13 21	1 3 5 11 13	1 3 11 13 16 21	1 2 11 13 16 21	1 3 5 11 13 16	1 11 13 16	DF	CHI SQ. VALUE	REF.
HILL TRIBES														
KAREN	39	O.	0	0	1	1	33	0	0	4	0	0		139
		E.	0.0	0.0	0.9	0.9	33.2	0.1	0.1	3.7	0.1			
LAHU	72	O.	2	0	18	9	42	1	0	0	0	1	1.730	139
		E.	1.8	1.7	17.7	6.9	42.8	0.2	0.1	0.8	0.0			
LISU	26	O.	2	1	1	5	10	1	2	3	1	4	7.345	139
		E.	0.4	1.7	3.7	4.7	8.1	1.0	1.3	4.5	0.6			
MEO	111	O.	5	0	36	8	58	0	0	4	0	3	4.161	139
		E.	4.8	1.8	34.0	5.9	60.6	0.8	0.1	3.0	0.0			
THAIS *														
CENTRAL	127	O.	3	1	16	13	91	0	0	3	0	2	2.557	139
		E.	1.0	1.7	19.2	12.0	90.1	0.3	0.2	2.5	0.0			
NORTH	148	O.	0	0	6	6	131	0	0	5	0	0		139
		E.	0.1	0.2	5.7	5.7	131.5	0.1	0.1	4.7	0.0			
NORTHEAST	196	O.	0	1	3	9	180	0	0	3	0	0		139
		E.	0.0	0.2	3.2	10.1	179.4	0.0	0.1	2.9	0.0			
SOUTH	153	O.	1	2	19	19	104	0	0	8	0	2	1.630	139
		E.	0.8	2.3	18.5	18.0	105.4	0.6	0.6	6.6	0.1			

* THREE SAMPLES SHOWED BLACK ADMIXTURE [GM(1,2,5,11,13,21), GM(1,5,11,13,21), AND GM(1,3,5,6,11,13,21)] AND ONE SAMPLE WAS GM(1,2,3,5,11,13). THE REGION(S) FROM WHICH THESE SAMPLES CAME FROM WAS NOT STATED.

HAPLOTYPES

MONGOLOIDS

ASIA

THAILAND	TOTAL		1 21	1 2 21	1 3 5 11 13	1 11 13 16	REF.
HILL TRIBES							
KAREN	39	F.	0.013	0.013	0.923	0.051	139
		S.E.	0.013	0.013	0.030	0.025	
LAHU	72	F.	0.160	0.063	0.771	0.007	139
		S.E.	0.031	0.020	0.035	0.007	
LISU	26	F.	0.127	0.161	0.558	0.154	139
		S.E.	0.048	0.053	0.069	0.050	
MEO	111	F.	0.207	0.036	0.739	0.018	139
		S.E.	0.027	0.013	0.029	0.009	
THAIS							
CENTRAL	127	F.	0.090	0.056	0.843	0.012	139
		S.E.	0.018	0.015	0.023	0.007	
NORTH	148	F.	0.020	0.020	0.943	0.017	139
		S.E.	0.008	0.008	0.014	0.007	
NORTHEAST	196	F.	0.009	0.027	0.957	0.008	139
		S.E.	0.005	0.008	0.010	0.004	
SOUTH	153	F.	0.073	0.071	0.830	0.026	139
		S.E.	0.015	0.015	0.021	0.009	

TABLE VIII-22
TESTED FOR GM 1, 2, 3, 5, 10, 11, 13, 14, 21, 23

PHENOTYPES

MONGOLOIDS
S. AMERICA
FRENCH GUIANA

			TOTAL	21	1 21	1 10 13 21	1 2 10 11 13 21	1 10 11 13	1 5 10 13 14 21	1 2 5 10 11 13 14 21	1 5 10 11 13 14	CHI SQ. DF	CHI SQ. VALUE	REF.
EMERILLON INDIANS	38	O.		17	7	11	1	0	1	1	0	2	1.436	21
		E.		18.1	7.2	8.3	1.5	0.9	1.4	0.3	0.3			
OYAMPI INDIANS OYAPOK	99	O.		63	25	8	2	1				1	0.609	21
		E.		62.1	25.2	9.5	1.8	0.4						
WAYANA INDIANS MARONI	165	O.		91	68	5	1	0				1	0.223	21
		E.		91.4	67.6	4.5	1.4	0.1						

HAPLOTYPES

MONGOLOIDS
S. AMERICA
FRENCH GUIANA

			TOTAL	21	1 21	1 2 21	1 10 11 13	1 5 10 11 13 14	REF.
EMERILLON INDIANS	38	F.		0.690	0.126	0.158	0.026		21
		S.E.		0.054	0.039	0.042	0.018		
OYAMPI INDIANS OYAPOK	99	F.		0.792	0.147	0.061			21
		S.E.		0.030	0.026	0.017			
WAYANA INDIANS MARONI	165	F.		0.744	0.237	0.018			21
		S.E.		0.026	0.025	0.007			

TABLE VIII-23
TESTED FOR GM 1, 2, 3, 5, 6, 11, 13, 15, 16, 21, 24

PHENOTYPES

MONGOLOIDS
S. AMERICA
SURINAM

	TOTAL	1 21 21	1 2 21	1 13 15 16 21	1 2 11 13 15 16 21	1 11 13 15 16		CHI SQ. DF	VALUE
TRIO INDIANS	376	O. 153	198	16	8	1		1	0.021
		E. 152.9	197.6	16.6	8.5	0.4			
WAJANA INDIANS	192	O. 107	79	5	1	0		1	0.216
		E. 107.4	78.6	4.5	1.4	0.0			

HAPLOTYPES

	21	1 21	1 2 21	1 13 15 16	REF.
	F. 0.638	0.328	0.035		37
	S.E. 0.019	0.019	0.007		
	F. 0.748	0.236	0.016		37
	S.E. 0.024	0.023	0.006		

TABLE VIII-24
TESTED FOR GM 1, 2, 3, 5, 11, 13, 15, 16, 17, 21, 23

PHENOTYPES

MONGOLOIDS
ASIA
TAIWAN

		1 7 2 1	1 2 17 21	1 3 5 11 13 17 21 23	1 3 5 11 13 17 21 23	1 2 3 5 11 13 17 21 23	1 3 5 11 13 17 21 23	1 2 3 5 11 13 17 21 23	1 3 5 11 13 21 23	1 3 21 23	CHI SQ. DF VALUE	REF.
TOTAL												
ABORIGINES	300 O.	9	7	95	18	170	1	0	0	0	1 1.327	81
	E.	12.1	5.7	90.8	19.4	171.0	0.2	0.0	0.8	0.0		

HAPLOTYPES

MONGOLOIDS
ASIA
TAIWAN

		1 7 2 1	1 2 17 21	1 3 5 11 13 23	1 3 21 23	REF.
TOTAL						
ABORIGINES	300 F.	0.201	0.043	0.755	0.002	81
	S.E.	0.016	0.008	0.018	0.002	

133

TABLE VIII-25
TESTED FOR GM 1, 2, 3, 5, 6, 11, 13, 14, 15, 16, 21, 24

PHENOTYPES

	TOTAL	1 21	1 2 21	1 3 5 11 13 14 21	1 3 5 11 13 14 21	1 3 11 13 15 16 21	1 2 11 13 15 16 21	1 3 5 11 13 15 16 21	1 3 5 11 14 16 21	1 3 5 11 13 14 15 16	CHI SQ. DF	VALUE	REF.
MONGOLOIDS													
ASIA													
JAPAN													
JAPANESE O.	100	22	17	7	3	1	28	11	4	7	4	0.798	69
JAPANESE E.		21.8	18.5	7.5	2.7	0.6	26.6	9.6	4.6	8.1			

HAPLOTYPES

	TOTAL	1 21	1 2 21	1 3 5 11 13 14	1 3 11 13 15 16	REF.
MONGOLOIDS						
ASIA						
JAPAN						
JAPANESE F.	100	0.467	0.168	0.080	0.285	69
JAPANESE S.E.		0.036	0.028	0.019	0.032	

TABLE VIII-26
TESTED FOR GM 1, 2, 3, 5, 6, 11, 13, 15, 16, 17, 21, 23, 24

PHENOTYPES

		17 21	1 17 21	13 21	1 3 5 11 13 17 21 23	1 2 3 5 11 13 17 21 23	1 3 5 11 13 15 16 17 21 23	1 2 3 5 11 13 15 16 17 21	1 3 5 11 13 15 16 17 23	1 3 5 11 13 15 16 17		CHI SQ.	
	TOTAL										DF	VALUE	REF.
MONGOLOIDS ASIA JAPAN													
JAPANESE OSAKA *	92 O.	16	13	13	3	2	19	12	8	6	5	2.931	70
	E.	15.2	14.7	11.4	4.6	2.1	20.7	8.4	7.8	7.1			

HAPLOTYPES

		1 17 21	1 2 17 21	1 3 5 11 13 23	1 3 11 13 15 16 17		
	TOTAL						REF.
MONGOLOIDS ASIA JAPAN							
JAPANESE OSAKA	92 F.	0.407	0.164	0.152	0.277		70
	S.E.	0.037	0.029	0.026	0.033		

* EXCLUDING ONE GM(1, 3, 11, 13, 15, 16, 17, 21, 23) SAMPLE.

135

TABLE VIII-27
TESTED FOR GM 1, 2, 3, 5, 6, 10, 11, 13, 15, 16, 17, 21, 23, 24

MONGOLOIDS

ASIA

THAILAND

THAIS   REF.   72

PHENOTYPES *

OBS.	EXP.	
3	1.5	1 , 17, 21
3	2.6	1 , 2, 17, 21
25	27.7	1 , 3, 5, 10, 11, 13, 17, 21, 23
18	18.4	1 , 2, 3, 5, 10, 11, 13, 17, 21, 23
130	129.3	1 , 3, 5, 10, 11, 13, 23
1	0.9	1 , 10, 11, 13, 15, 16, 17, 21
1	0.6	1 , 2, 10, 11, 13, 15, 16, 17, 21
8	8.0	1 , 3, 5, 10, 11, 13, 15, 16, 17, 23
0	0.1	1 , 10, 11, 13, 15, 16, 17
0	0.5	1 , 5, 10, 11, 13, 17, 21
0	0.6	1 , 2, 5, 10, 11, 13, 17, 23
5	4.8	1 , 5, 10, 11, 13, 15, 16, 17
0	0.2	1 , 5, 10, 11, 13, 15, 16, 17
0	0.0	1 , 5, 10, 11, 13, 17
2	1.6	1 , 2, 3, 5, 10, 11, 13, 17, 23
0	0.1	1 , 2, 5, 10, 11, 13, 15, 16, 17
0	0.3	1 , 3, 5, 10, 11, 13, 17
0	0.2	1 , 3, 17, 21
2	2.4	1 , 3, 5, 10, 11, 13, 21, 23
0	0.1	1 , 3, 10, 11, 13, 15, 16, 17, 21
0	0.0	1 , 3, 5, 10, 11, 13, 17, 21
0	0.0	1 , 2, 5, 10, 211, 13, 17, 21
0	0.0	1 , 3, 21

TOTAL 198   198.0

CHI SQUARE= 1.873   D.F. = 4

HAPLOTYPES

FREQ.	S.E.	
0.086	0.014	1 , 17, 21
0.057	0.012	1 , 2, 17, 21
0.808	0.020	1 , 3, 5, 10, 11, 13, 23
0.025	0.008	1 , 10, 11, 13, 15, 16, 17
0.013	0.006	1 , 5, 10, 11, 13, 17
0.005	0.004	1 , 2, 5, 10, 11, 13, 17
0.005	0.004	1 , 3, 21

* EXCLUDING ONE GM(1,2,17,21,23) SAMPLE.

136

TABLE IX-1

TABLE IX-1
TESTED FOR GM 1, 2, 5

PHENOTYPES

NEGROIDS AFRICA ALGERIA	TOTAL		1 5	1 2 5	1 2	5	1	CHI SQ. DF	VALUE
HARRATIN HOGGAR MTS.	207	O. E.	205 205.0	1 0.9	0 0.1		1 1.0	0	
SENEGAL									
BASSARI	25	O. E.	25					0	
BEDIK	165	O. E.	161 161.1	1 0.9	0 0.1		3 2.9	0	
DAKAR									
OUOLOF	164	O. E.	164					0	
PEULH	94	O. E.	94					0	
SERERES	118	O. E.	118					0	
TOUCOULEUR	57	O. E.	57					0	

HAPLOTYPES

		1 5	1 2	1 5	1	REF.
HARRATIN HOGGAR MTS.	F. S.E.	0.929 0.034	0.002 0.002		0.068 0.034	6
BASSARI	F. S.E.	1.000				38
BEDIK	F. S.E.	0.864 0.038	0.003 0.003		0.133 0.038	38
OUOLOF	F. S.E.	1.000				123
PEULH	F. S.E.	1.000				123
SERERES	F. S.E.	1.000				123
TOUCOULEUR	F. S.E.	1.000				123

137

TABLE IX-1 CONTINUED
TESTED FOR GM 1, 2, 5

PHENOTYPES

	TOTAL		1 5	1 2 5	1 2	CHI SQ. DF	VALUE
NEGROIDS							
AFRICA							
UPPER VOLTA							
MARKA	166	O.	162	4	0	0	
		E.	162.0	4.0	0.0		
PEULH	111	O.	111			0	
		E.					
W. AFRICA							
BASSARI	120	O.	120			0	
		E.					
CONIAGUI	53	O.	53			0	
		E.					
N. AMERICA							
U.S.A.							
OAKLAND, CA.	260	O.	239	8	2 8 3	1	0.554
		E.	238.6	8.8	1.3 8.0 3.4		

HAPLOTYPES

		1 5	1 2	5	1	REF.
MARKA	F.	0.988	0.012			198
	S.E.	0.006	0.006			
PEULH	F.	1.000				198
	S.E.					
BASSARI	F.	1.000				39
	S.E.					
CONIAGUI	F.	1.000				39
	S.E.					
OAKLAND, CA.	F.	0.691	0.020	0.175	0.114	106
	S.E.	0.042	0.006	0.031	0.030	

TABLE IX-2
TESTED FOR GM 1, 2, 3, 5

PHENOTYPES

	TOTAL		1 5	1 2 5	1 3 5	1 2 3 5	3 5	1	CHI SQ. DF	VALUE
NEGROIDS										
NORTH AMERICA										
U.S.A.										
BOSTON, MA.	67	O.	46	4	0	15	0	1	1	0.528
		E.	46.9	3.7	0.6	13.5	1.0	0.7		

HAPLOTYPES

		1 5	1 2	3 5	1	REF.
BOSTON, MA.	F.	0.739	0.037	0.119	0.104	67
	S.E.	0.062	0.017	0.028	0.056	

138

TABLE IX-3
TESTED FOR GM 1, 2, 5, 6

NEGROIDS

AFRICA

PHENOTYPES

CAMEROUN	TOTAL		1 5	1 5 6	1 2 5	1 2 5 6	1 2	5	1	CHI SQ. DF	VALUE
BAMILEKES	60	O.	28	23	0	9	0			1	18.990
		E.	23.1	28.2	5.6	2.7	0.3				
′ OMITTING GM(2)	60	O.	28	32						0	
		E.	28.0	32.0							
CONGO											
BASHI BAKAVU	37	O.	17	18					2	0	
		E.	17.0	18.0					2.0		
PYGMIES ITURI FOREST	120	O.	113	7						0	
		E.	113.0	7.0							
DAHOMEY											
PORTO-NOVO	100	O.	59	41						0	
		E.	59.0	41.0							
MADAGASCAR											
TANANARIVE	159	O.	131	28						0	
		E.	131.0	28.0							
NIGERIA											
YORUBU IBADAN	35	O.	17	18						0	
		E.	17.0	18.0							
FULANI NORTH REGION	35	O.	19	16						0	
		E.	19.0	16.0							

HAPLOTYPES

CAMEROUN		1 5	1 5 6	1 5 2	5	1	REF.
BAMILEKES	F.	0.621	0.304	0.075			27
	S.E.	0.048	0.046	0.024			
′ OMITTING GM(2)	F.	0.683	0.317				
	S.E.	0.047	0.047				
BASHI BAKAVU	F.	0.484	0.283			0.232	162
	S.E.	0.087	0.057			0.080	
PYGMIES ITURI FOREST	F.	0.970	0.030				162
	S.E.	0.011	0.011				
PORTO-NOVO	F.	0.768	0.232				27
	S.E.	0.032	0.032				
TANANARIVE	F.	0.908	0.092				27
	S.E.	0.017	0.017				
YORUBU IBADAN	F.	0.697	0.303				162
	S.E.	0.061	0.061				
FULANI NORTH REGION	F.	0.737	0.263				162
	S.E.	0.057	0.057				

139

TABLE IX-3 CONTINUED
TESTED FOR GM 1,2,5,6

NEGROIDS

AFRICA

SENEGAL

	TOTAL		PHENOTYPES 1 5	1 5 6	1 2 5	1 2 5 6	1 2	5	1	CHI SQ. DF	VALUE	HAPLOTYPES 1 5	1 5 6	1 2	5	1	REF.
DAKAR *	398	O.	136	262													114
		E.	136.0	262.0						0							
		F.										0.585	0.415				
		S.E.										0.020	0.020				

UPPER VOLTA

	TOTAL		1 5	1 5 6	1 2 5	1 2 5 6	1 2	5	1	DF	VALUE	1 5	1 5 6	1 2	5	1	REF.
TRIBE NOT STATED #	245	O.	140	104					1								27
		E.	140.0	104.0					1.0	0							
		F.										0.695	0.241			0.064	
		S.E.										0.037	0.021			0.032	

C. AMERICA

MARTINIQUE

	TOTAL		1 5	1 5 6	1 2 5	1 2 5 6	1 2	5	1	DF	VALUE	1 5	1 5 6	1 2	5	1	REF.
FORT-DE-FRANCE #	299	O.	196	78	17	1	0	7									27
		E.	197.7	76.6	14.9	2.6	0.3	7.1		1	1.527						
		F.										0.674	0.142	0.030	0.154		
		S.E.										0.031	0.015	0.007	0.029		

N. AMERICA

U.S.A.

	TOTAL		1 5	1 5 6	1 2 5	1 2 5 6	1 2	5	1	DF	VALUE	1 5	1 5 6	1 2	5	1	REF.
CLAXTON, GA.	189	O.	113	74	1	0	0	1									10
		E.	113.2	73.8	0.7	0.2	0.1	1.0		0							
		F.										0.706	0.220	0.003	0.003	0.071	
		S.E.										0.041	0.023	0.003	0.036	
CLEVELAND, OH.	364	O.	240	98	7	3	1	7	8								153
		E.	239.1	99.2	7.6	1.7	1.7	7.0	7.7	2	1.455						
		F.										0.551	0.150	0.015	0.138	0.146	
		S.E.										0.037	0.014	0.005	0.026	0.025	
CLEVELAND, OH.	317	O.	203	95	5	3	2	6	3								154
		E.	201.3	96.2	7.2	1.7	1.2	5.9	3.5	2	2.380						
		F.										0.573	0.169	0.016	0.137	0.105	
		S.E.										0.040	0.016	0.005	0.028	0.027	

* EXCLUDING ONE GM(1,2,5) AND ONE GM(1,2,5,6) SAMPLES.

EXCLUDING ONE GM(5,6) SAMPLE.

TABLE IX-4
TESTED FOR GM 1, 2, 3, 5, 6

PHENOTYPES

NEGROIDS

NORTH AMERICA

U.S.A.

		1 5	1 5 6	1 2 5	1 2 5 6	1 2 1 2	1 3 5	1 3 5 6	1 2 3 5	3 5	1	DF	CHI SQ. VALUE	REF.
CLEVELAND, OH.	186 O.	91	46	4	0	1	27	8	2	4	3			
	E.	88.8	45.8	4.1	1.1	1.0	31.6	7.1	0.9	2.7	3.0	4	3.335	156

HAPLOTYPES

NEGROIDS

NORTH AMERICA

U.S.A.

		1 5	1 5 6	1 2	1 3 5	1	REF.
CLEVELAND, OH.	186 F.	0.576	0.158	0.019	0.121	0.126	
	S.E.	0.040	0.020	0.007	0.017	0.035	156

141

TABLE IX-5
TESTED FOR GM 1, 2, 3, 5, 10

PHENOTYPES

	TOTAL		1 5 10	1 5	1	1 3 5 10	3 5 10	DF	CHI SQ. VALUE
NEGROIDS									
AFRICA									
KENYA									
CENTRAL NYANZA DISTRICT	366	O.	336	20	2	8			
		E.	336.0	20.0	2.0	8.0	0	0	
		E.	336.0	20.0	2.0	7.9	0.0	0	

HAPLOTYPES

	1 5 10	1 5	1 5 1	1 3 5 10	1 3 5	3 5 10	REF.
F.	0.744	0.171	0.074	0.011			53
S.E.	0.025	0.031	0.026	0.004			
F.	0.744	0.171	0.074	0.011			
S.E.	0.025	0.031	0.026	0.004			

TABLE IX-6
TESTED FOR GM 3, 5, 11, 13, 14

PHENOTYPES

	TOTAL		5 11 13 14	5 11	DF	CHI SQ. VALUE
NEGROIDS						
AFRICA						
IVORY COAST						
BAOULES	487	O.	452	35		
		E.	452.0	35.0	0	
YAOURES	227	O.	216	11		
		E.	216.0	11.0	0	
SENEGAL						
BANAPAS	378	O.	360	18		
		E.	360.0	18.0	0	
BIWOLS	360	O.	341	19		
		E.	341.0	19.0	0	

HAPLOTYPES

		5 11 13 14	5 11	REF.
BAOULES	F.	0.732	0.268	9
	S.E.	0.022	0.022	
YAOURES	F.	0.780	0.220	9
	S.E.	0.032	0.032	
BANAPAS	F.	0.782	0.218	9
	S.E.	0.025	0.025	
BIWOLS	F.	0.770	0.230	9
	S.E.	0.026	0.026	

TABLE IX—7
TESTED FOR GM 1, 2, 3, 5, 11, 13

NEGROIDS
AFRICA
TANZANIA

PHENOTYPES

	TOTAL		1 5 11 13	1 2 5 11 13	1 2	1 3 5 11 13	1 2 3 5 11 13	3 5 11 13	DF	CHI SQ. VALUE
NYATURA	67	O.	64	1	0	2	0	0	0	0
		E.	64.0	1.0	0.0	2.0	0.0	0.0		
SANDAWE	176	O.	170	3	0	3	0	0	0	0
		E.	170.1	2.9	0.0	2.9	0.0	0.0		

HAPLOTYPES

		1 5 11 13	1 2	3 5 11 13	REF.
NYATURA	F.	0.978	0.007	0.015	42
	S.E.	0.013	0.007	0.010	
SANDAWE	F.	0.983	0.009	0.009	42
	S.E.	0.007	0.005	0.005	

143

TABLE IX-8
TESTED FOR GM 1, 2, 3, 5, 6, 11, 13

PHENOTYPES

		1 5 6 11 13	1 5 6 11 13	1 5 6 11	1 5 11 13	1 2 5 11 13	1 2 5 6 11	1 2 11 13	1 2 5 6 11 13	1 (3) 5 6 11 13	1 2 (3) 5 11 13	1 2 (3) 5 6 11 13	1	1 2 (3) 5 6 11 13	DF	CHI SQ. VALUE	REF.
NEGROIDS																	
AFRICA																	
CENTRAL AFRICAN EMPIRE TOTAL																	
BABINGA PYGMIES 162	O.	119	38	5											1	0.809	16
	E.	117.6	40.9	3.6													
3. AMERICA																	
SURINAM																	
PARAMARIBO REGION * 125	O.	52	29	7	3	0	1	1	7.8	13	2	4	2	4	2	51.900	69
	E.	54.3	22.9	9.9	1.7	0.0	6.1	1.5	7.8	15.8	3.9	1.2	1.1	2.7	6	18.019	
	E.	47.8	27.3	6.5	2.8	5.5	1.3	0.6	3.5	15.6	4.1	1.3	1.1	2.6	4	13.790	
	E.	48.5	29.6	4.2	2.3	0.0	2.0	1.2	8.6	15.5	4.1	1.3	1.1	6.3			
' OMITTING GM(2) 125	O.	52	30	8	3					17	2		2	11	3	18.430	
	E.	59.9	21.8	12.2	3.5					12.2	8.7		1.1	5.7	2	1.991	
	E.	52.7	28.5	7.6	3.0					16.8	4.1		1.1	11.2			
NON-PARAMARIBO REGIONS * 883	O.	396	347	90	17	13	1	1	2.4	3	1	0	2	2	4	10.356	69
	E.	399.6	335.0	97.6	17.3	15.6	0.9	0.9	0.4	5.5	0.1	0.0	1.5	4.7	5	26.992	
	E.	387.6	362.6	80.4	15.9	12.7	1.9	5.7	1.9	5.4	0.1	0.0	4.6	1.5	3	8.200	
	E.	392.5	349.2	89.4	17.1	15.4	0.8	2.4	0.5	5.5	0.1	0.0	2.8	4.9			
' OMITTING GM(2) 883	O.	409	353	91	18					4	4	0	4	2	2	4.166	
	E.	416.8	336.5	101.1	18.3					5.2	2.7	0.0	2.2	2.2			

* ALL SAMPLES WERE TESTED FOR GM(13).   SELECTED SAMPLES (NOT SPECIFIED) WERE TESTED FOR GM(10).

HAPLOTYPES

			1 5 1 3	1 5 6 11	1 1 3	1 2	3 5 1 3	1 1 1 3	1	1 2 5 11 13	1 5 6 11 13	REF

NEGROIDS

AFRICA

CENTRAL AFRICAN EMPIRE
  TOTAL

			1 5 1 3	1 5 6 11	1 1 3	1 2	3 5 1 3	1 1 1 3	1	1 2 5 11 13	1 5 6 11 13	REF
BABINGA PYGMIES	162	F.	0.832	0.148								16
		S.E.	0.020	0.020								

3. AMERICA

SURINAM

			1 5 1 3	1 5 6 11	1 1 3	1 2	3 5 1 3	1 1 1 3	1	1 2 5 11 13	1 5 6 11 13	REF
PARAMARIBO REGION	125	F.	0.497	0.170	0.042	0.143	0.092	0.147	0.091			69
		S.E.	0.046	0.053	0.022	0.039	0.017	0.086	0.032			
		F.	0.403	0.094	0.044	0.055	0.092	0.230			0.083	
		S.E.	0.042	0.030	0.023	0.015	0.018	0.040			0.030	
		F.	0.414	0.066	0.039	0.121	0.092	0.224	0.065		0.111	
		S.E.	0.045	0.019	0.020	0.039	0.018	0.043	0.023		0.023	
' OMITTING GM(2)	125	F.	0.473	0.164	0.057		0.092	0.214				
		S.E.	0.040	0.025	0.028		0.018	0.036				
		F.	0.395	0.089	0.036		0.092	0.299			0.088	
		S.E.	0.043	0.030	0.021		0.018	0.043			0.030	
NON-PARAMARIBO REGIONS	883	F.	0.542	0.293	0.104	0.005	0.005	0.042	0.009			69
		S.E.	0.018	0.011	0.018	0.002	0.002	0.012	0.003			
		F.	0.527	0.238	0.080	0.014	0.005	0.072			0.064	
		S.E.	0.018	0.019	0.016	0.003	0.002	0.015			0.019	
		F.	0.533	0.267	0.093	0.005	0.005	0.057	0.009		0.032	
		S.E.	0.019	0.021	0.018	0.002	0.002	0.016	0.003		0.021	
' OMITTING GM(2)	883	F.	0.551	0.292	0.102		0.005	0.050				
		S.E.	0.018	0.011	0.018		0.002	0.013				
		F.	0.540	0.261	0.090		0.005	0.067			0.037	
		S.E.	0.019	0.021	0.018		0.002	0.017			0.021	

145

TABLE IX-9
TESTED FOR GM 1, 2, 3, 5, 6, 13, 14

PHENOTYPES

		TOTAL	1 5 13 14	1 5 6 13 14	1 5 6	1 5 6 14	1 5 6 13	1 13	1	1 3 5 13 14	1 3 5 6 13 14	3 5 13 14	1 5 14	DF	CHI SQ. VALUE	REF.
NEGROIDS																
AFRICA																
NEGROES	O.	106	50	47	4	5										158
	E.		51.0	45.1	4.4	5.5								1	0.194	
ANGOLA																
MIXED TRIBES	O.	111	73	30	5	3										64
	E.		69.8	36.5	3.0	1.8								1	3.492	
CHAD																
SARA MAJINGAY	O.	255	199	52	4											55
	E.		198.5	52.9	3.5									1	0.081	
BOTSWANA																
BECHUANA	O.	155	93	36	4	9	4	9					0			64
	E.		91.4	38.6	2.0	7.5	7.7	7.3					0.4	1	3.640	
	E.		88.4	44.6	1.8	5.3	7.4	7.6						2	9.146	
	E.		96.7	30.8	5.2	5.4	10.4	5.1					1.4	3	11.957	
NGALAGADI	O.	48	26	7	3	2	8	2					0			62
	E.		24.0	9.5	2.8	1.8	6.2	3.4					0.3	2	2.008	
LESOTHO																
BASUTU	O.	149	81	39	3	13	6	4	2	1	0					64
	E.		79.0	42.7	4.3	11.0	3.5	5.9	1.6	0.8	0.2	0.0		2	3.599	
	E.		79.0	42.7	4.3	11.0	3.5	5.9	1.6	0.8	0.2	0.0		2	3.649	
MALAWI																
MIXED TRIBES	O.	153	69	64	7	7	2	1	2	2	1	0				64
	E.		70.3	61.4	7.0	7.7	3.2	0.4	2.0	0.9	0.9	0.0		2	1.006	
	E.		70.3	61.4	7.0	7.7	3.2	0.4	2.1	0.9	0.9	0.0		2	1.022	

HAPLOTYPES

NEGROIDS

AFRICA

	TOTAL		1/5/13/14	1/5/6	1/5/6/14	1/13	3/5/13/14	1/3/5/13/14	1/5/14	REF.
NEGROES	106	F.	0.693	0.204	0.102					158
		S.E.	0.032	0.042	0.038					

ANGOLA

			1/5/13/14	1/5/6	1/5/6/14	1/13	3/5/13/14	1/3/5/13/14	1/5/14	REF.
MIXED TRIBES	111	F.	0.793	0.164	0.043					64
		S.E.	0.027	0.036	0.030					

CHAD

			1/5/13/14	1/5/6	1/5/6/14	1/13	3/5/13/14	1/3/5/13/14	1/5/14	REF.
SARA MAJINGAY	255	F.	0.882	0.118						55
		S.E.	0.014	0.014						

BOTSWANA

			1/5/13/14	1/5/6	1/5/6/14	1/13	3/5/13/14	1/3/5/13/14	1/5/14	REF.
BECHUANA	155	F.	0.530	0.114	0.086	0.217			0.053	64
		S.E.	0.045	0.030	0.030	0.037			0.030	
		F.	0.565	0.107	0.106	0.222			0.095	
		S.E.	0.040	0.029	0.029	0.037			0.028	
		F.	0.539	0.184		0.182				
		S.E.	0.042	0.022		0.031				
NGALAGADI		F.	0.413	0.240		0.268			0.079	62
		S.E.	0.068	0.044		0.055			0.044	

LESOTHO

			1/5/13/14	1/5/6	1/5/6/14	1/13	3/5/13/14	1/3/5/13/14	1/5/14	REF.
BASUTU	149	F.	0.538	0.097	0.138	0.121	0.102	0.003		64
		S.E.	0.039	0.029	0.030	0.035	0.031	0.003		
		F.	0.538	0.097	0.138	0.121	0.102	0.003		
		S.E.	0.039	0.029	0.030	0.035	0.031	0.003		

MALAWI

			1/5/13/14	1/5/6	1/5/6/14	1/13	3/5/13/14	1/3/5/13/14	1/5/14	REF.
MIXED TRIBES	153	F.	0.631	0.214	0.096	0.048		0.010		64
		S.E.	0.034	0.034	0.030	0.023		0.006		
		F.	0.631	0.214	0.096	0.048		0.010		
		S.E.	0.034	0.034	0.030	0.023		0.006		

TABLE IX-9 CONTINUED
TESTED FOR GM 1, 2, 3, 5, 6, 13, 14

PHENOTYPES

NEGROIDS
AFRICA
MOZAMBIQUE

	TOTAL		1 5 13 14	1 5 6 13 14	1 5 6	1 5 6 14	1 5 6 13	1 5 13	1	1 3 5 13 14	1 3 5 6 13 14	3 5 13 14	1 5 14	DF	CHI SQ. VALUE	REF.
NYAMBAAN	119	O.	69	37	6	6	1	1	0				0	0		
		E.	67.5	39.8	5.2	5.2	1.0	1.0	0.0				0.4	1	3.524	64
		E.	65.0	44.8	4.1	4.0	1.0	0.1	0.0					1	0.873	
		E.	68.8	37.4	6.6	4.5	0.9	0.9	0.0				0.8			
SHANGAAN * TONGA	152	O.	73	67	2	7	2	1						1	2.142	64
		E.	76.8	59.6	2.3	10.1	2.5	0.6								
SOUTH AFRICA																
BACA	137	O.	67	41	4	10	8	6		1	0	0		2	0.172	64
		E.	67.0	41.2	3.5	9.8	8.9	5.6		0.7	0.3	0.0		2	1.748	
		E.	64.2	46.4	3.2	7.6	8.7	5.9		0.7	0.3					
HLUBI #	145	O.	78	43	2	8	2	9	3					2	2.110	64
		E.	80.7	38.1	2.1	11.0	2.3	8.9	2.0							
NDEBELE TRANSVAAL @	103	O.	50	43	4	5	1	0	0	1	0	0		0		64
		E.	50.3	42.4	4.2	5.2	0.9	0.0	0.0	0.7	0.3	0.0				
PEDI $	146	O.	65	54	0	18	5	2	1	1	0	0		1	5.578	64
		E.	64.2	55.8	1.7	16.9	2.5	3.6	0.3	0.7	0.3	0.0		1	5.574	
		E.	64.2	55.8	1.7	16.9	2.5	3.6	0.3	0.7	0.3					
PONDO %	112	O.	53	32	2	16	5	4					0	1	1.130	64
		E.	50.6	36.0	1.8	13.6	5.3	3.9					0.8	2	7.420	
		E.	46.8	44.0	1.7	10.2	5.2	4.1						3	16.857	
		E.	57.5	26.0	7.3	8.9	7.6	2.0					2.7			

* EXCLUDING ONE GM(1,5,14) SAMPLE.

EXCLUDING ONE GM(1,5) AND ONE GM(1,2,3,5,13,14) SAMPLES.

@ EXCLUDING ONE GM(5,6,13,14) AND ONE GM(1,2,5,13,14) SAMPLES.

$ EXCLUDING ONE GM(5,13,14) SAMPLE.

% EXCLUDING ONE GM(1,2,5,13,14) SAMPLE.

HAPLOTYPES

NEGROIDS
AFRICA

	TOTAL		1 5 13 14	1 5 6	1 5 6 14	1 13	1	3 5 13 14	1 3 5 13 14	1 5 14	REF.
MOZAMBIQUE											
NYAMBAAN	119	F.	0.680	0.209	0.036	0.020				0.056	64
		S.E.	0.041	0.041	0.040	0.018				0.035	
		F.	0.716	0.185	0.076	0.024				0.080	
		S.E.	0.034	0.038	0.033	0.021				0.028	
		F.	0.667	0.235		0.017					
		S.E.	0.040	0.027		0.016					
SHANGAAN TONGA	152	F.	0.648	0.124	0.162	0.065					64
		S.E.	0.038	0.036	0.038	0.030					
SOUTH AFRICA											
BACA	137	F.	0.482	0.160	0.152	0.202		0.004			64
		S.E.	0.046	0.032	0.039	0.034		0.004			
		F.	0.508	0.152	0.129	0.208			0.004		
		S.E.	0.041	0.034	0.033	0.037			0.004		
HLUBI	145	F.	0.521	0.050	0.155	0.157	0.117				64
		S.E.	0.040	0.023	0.028	0.039	0.033				
NDEBELE TRANSVAAL	103	F.	0.677	0.201	0.100	0.022					64
		S.E.	0.037	0.042	0.038	0.021					
PEDI	146	F.	0.519	0.071	0.242	0.118	0.047	0.003			64
		S.E.	0.042	0.031	0.036	0.039	0.029	0.003			
		F.	0.519	0.071	0.242	0.118	0.047		0.003		
		S.E.	0.042	0.031	0.036	0.039	0.029		0.003		
PONDO	112	F.	0.433	0.127	0.170	0.188				0.082	64
		S.E.	0.052	0.037	0.042	0.042				0.035	
		F.	0.483	0.172	0.204	0.191				0.156	
		S.E.	0.047	0.037	0.040	0.043				0.033	
		F.	0.456	0.254		0.133					
		S.E.	0.046	0.029		0.032					

TABLE IX-9 CONTINUED
GM 1, 2, 3, 5, 6, 13, 14 TESTED FOR

PHENOTYPES

NEGROIDS		TOTAL	1 5 6 13 14	1 5 6 13 14	1 5 6	1 5 6 14	1 5 6 13	1 5 13	1	1 3 5 13 14	1 3 5 6 13 14	3 5 13 14	DF	CHI SQ. VALUE	REF.
AFRICA															
SOUTH AFRICA															
SWAZI	O.	126	62	49	2	6	5	1		0	0				
	E.		62.9	46.7	2.9	7.1	4.0	1.4		0.7	0.7		1	0.877	64
	E.		62.9	46.7	2.9	7.1	4.0	1.4		0.7	0.3	0.0	1	0.877	
VENDA	O.	80	38	31	2	5	1	3							
	E.		38.6	29.8	1.1	5.5	2.9	2.0					2	2.671	64
XHOSA	O.	214	110	48	6	11	8	26	2	2	1	0			
	E.		109.9	48.0	5.3	11.2	9.1	25.3	2.4	2.4	0.6	0.0	2	0.328	64
	E.		109.9	48.0	5.3	11.2	9.1	25.3	2.4	2.4	0.6	0.0	2	0.334	
ZULU *	O.	130	61	43	4	10	7	5							
	E.		59.0	46.7	3.3	8.4	7.9	4.7					2	0.934	64
S. W. AFRICA															
OKAVANGO															
BUNJA	O.	111	45	50	2	12	1	0		1	0	0			
	E.		45.3	49.7	2.1	12.0	0.8	0.1		0.6	0.4	0.0	0		64
	E.		45.3	49.7	2.1	12.0	0.8	0.1		0.6	0.4	0.0	0		
DIRIKO	O.	59	25	24	7	1			1	1	0	0			
	E.		26.6	21.5	8.2	1.2			0.6	0.7	0.3	0.0	0		64
	E.		26.6	21.5	8.2	1.2			0.6	0.7	0.3	0.0	0		
KUANGARI *	O.	46	24	17	1	3	1	0							
	E.		23.5	17.9	1.0	2.7	0.8	0.1					0		
MBUKUSHU	O.	115	52	53	2	7				0	1	0			
	E.		53.6	49.1	2.5	8.8			0.7	0.7	0.3	0.0	0		64
	E.		53.6	49.1	2.5	8.8			0.7	0.7	0.3	0.0	0		

* EXCLUDING ONE GM(1, 2, 5, 13, 14) SAMPLE.

HAPLOTYPES

NEGROIDS
AFRICA
SOUTH AFRICA

	TOTAL		1 5 13 14	1 5 6	1 5 14	1 13	1	3 5 13 14	1 3 5 13 14	REF.
SWAZI	126	F.	0.608	0.150	0.131	0.106		0.004	0.004	64
		S.E.	0.042	0.038	0.037	0.035		0.004	0.004	
		F.	0.608	0.150	0.131	0.106				
		S.E.	0.042	0.038	0.037	0.035				
VENDA	80	F.	0.554	0.116	0.171	0.158				64
		S.E.	0.056	0.045	0.047	0.050				
XHOSA	214	F.	0.442	0.083	0.108	0.254	0.105	0.007		64
		S.E.	0.031	0.020	0.020	0.034	0.027	0.004		
		F.	0.442	0.083	0.108	0.254	0.105			
		S.E.	0.031	0.020	0.020	0.034	0.027			
ZULU	130	F.	0.509	0.159	0.141	0.191				64
		S.E.	0.042	0.035	0.035	0.038				

S. W. AFRICA
OKAVANGO

	TOTAL		1 5 13 14	1 5 6	1 5 14	1 13	1	3 5 13 14	1 3 5 13 14	REF.
BUNJA	111	F.	0.612	0.137	0.219	0.027		0.005	0.005	64
		S.E.	0.040	0.045	0.048	0.026		0.004	0.005	
		F.	0.612	0.137	0.219	0.027				
		S.E.	0.040	0.045	0.048	0.026				
DIRIKO	59	F.	0.581	0.288	0.025		0.097	0.008	0.009	64
		S.E.	0.055	0.049	0.022		0.050	0.008	0.008	
		F.	0.581	0.288	0.025		0.097			
		S.E.	0.055	0.049	0.022		0.050			
KUANGARI	46	F.	0.662	0.148	0.134	0.055				64
		S.E.	0.066	0.066	0.065	0.049				
MBUKUSHU	115	F.	0.683	0.148	0.165			0.004	0.004	64
		S.E.	0.031	0.044	0.044			0.004	0.004	
		F.	0.683	0.148	0.165					
		S.E.	0.031	0.044	0.044					

TABLE IX-9   CONTINUED
TESTED FOR GM 1,2,3,5,6,13,14

PHENOTYPES

NEGROIDS AFRICA	TOTAL	1 5 13 14	1 5 6 13 14	1 5 6	1 5 6 14	1 5 6 13	1 5 13	1	1 3 5 13 14	1 3 5 6 13 14	3 5 13 14	DF	CHI SQ. VALUE	REF.
S.W. AFRICA														
OKAVANGO														
SAMBIO O.	98	40	42	4	10			2				0		64
E.		43.0	36.8	4.9	12.3			1.0						
OVAHIMBA KAOKOVELD O.	54	25	23	0	3	2	0					0		64
E.		26.3	20.8	0.6	3.9	1.0	0.5		0.7	0.3	0.0	0		
E.		26.3	20.8	0.6	3.9	1.0	0.5		0.7	0.3	0.0			
KUAMBI OVAMBOLAND O.	119	70	44	2	3							1	0.346	64
E.		71.1	41.7	2.5	3.7									
KUANYAMA OVAMBOLAND O.	118	57	54	2	4	1	0					0		64
E.		60.5	47.2	3.2	6.3	0.8	0.0							
ZAMBIA														
ILA KAFUE RIVER O.	41	22	19	0	0							0		64
E.		24.2	14.6	1.0	1.2							1	3.729	
E.		24.2	14.6	2.2								1	3.729	
E.		24.2	14.6		2.2									
LENJE O.	175	62	99	5	6	3	0					1	13.024	64
E.		72.8	77.9	10.1	11.9	2.2	0.1							
MLOZI ZAMBESI RIVER O.	189	100	63	7	15	4	0					1	4.368	64
E.		93.8	75.0	5.5	10.8	3.4	0.5							
PLATEAU TONGA O.	120	61	50	4	3	1	1					1	1.149	64
E.		63.5	45.2	4.6	4.2	2.2	0.3							
ZAMBESI VALLEY TONGA * O.	164	75	69	10	6	3	1					1	0.156	64
E.		76.1	67.0	10.1	6.4	4.1	0.4							

* EXCLUDING ONE GM(1,2,5,13,14) SAMPLE.

HAPLOTYPES

NEGROIDS

AFRICA

	TOTAL		1 5 13 14	1 5 6	1 5 6 14	1 13	1	3 5 13 14	1 3 5 13 14	REF.
S.W. AFRICA										
OKAVANGO										
SAMBIO	98	F.	0.569	0.145	0.185		0.101			64
		S.E.	0.043	0.045	0.042		0.039			
OVAHIMBA KAOKOVELD	54	F.	0.612	0.102	0.185	0.092		0.009		64
		S.E.	0.069	0.059	0.063	0.057		0.009		
		F.	0.611	0.102	0.185	0.092			0.009	
		S.E.	0.069	0.059	0.063	0.057			0.009	
KUAMBI OVAMBOLAND	119	F.	0.773	0.143	0.083					64
		S.E.	0.027	0.039	0.037					
KUANYAMA OVAMBOLAND	118	F.	0.696	0.165	0.119	0.020				64
		S.E.	0.035	0.041	0.039	0.021				
ZAMBIA										
ILA KAFUE RIVER	41	F.	0.768	0.154	0.078					64
		S.E.	0.047	0.066	0.060					
		F.	0.768	0.232						
		S.E.	0.047	0.047						
		F.	0.768		0.232					
		S.E.	0.047		0.047					
LENJE	175	F.	0.620	0.240	0.114	0.026				64
		S.E.	0.029	0.033	0.029	0.016				
MLOZI ZAMBESI RIVER	189	F.	0.653	0.170	0.124	0.053				64
		S.E.	0.032	0.032	0.031	0.023				
PLATEAU TONGA	120	F.	0.681	0.195	0.075	0.048				64
		S.E.	0.037	0.038	0.032	0.026				
ZAMBESI VALLEY TONGA	164	F.	0.633	0.248	0.069	0.050				64
		S.E.	0.032	0.031	0.025	0.021				

153

TABLE IX-10
TESTED FOR GM 1, 2, 3, 5, 6, 13, 14, 17, 21

PHENOTYPES

NEGROIDS
AFRICA
GAMBIA

	TOTAL		1 5 13 14 17	1 5 6 13 14 17	1 5 6 14 17	1 5 6 13 17	1 5 6 13 14 17 21	1 13 17 21	1 5 13 14 17 21	1 5 6 17 21	1 5 6 14 17 21	1 5 13 17 21	1 17 21	CHI SQ. DF	VALUE	REF.
KENEBA	822	O.	559	229	22	1	6	3	2	0	0	0	0	2	3.443	177
		E.	562.3	223.0	22.9	1.1	9.6	1.0	1.6	0.3	0.0	0.1	0.0			
MANDUAR	307	O.	228	69	4	2	4	0						1	0.432	177
		E.	227.3	70.3	4.1	1.8	3.0	0.5								

HAPLOTYPES

NEGROIDS
AFRICA
GAMBIA

	TOTAL		1 5 13 14 17	1 5 6 14 17	1 5 6 13 17	1 13 17 21	1 17 21	REF.
KENEBA	822	F.	0.793	0.167	0.004	0.035	0.001	177
		S.E.	0.013	0.010	0.004	0.009	0.001	
MANDUAR	307	F.	0.820	0.115	0.023	0.042		177
		S.E.	0.023	0.019	0.016	0.019		

TABLE IX-11
TESTED FOR GM 1, 2, 3, 5, 6, 11, 13, 14, 15, 16, 21, 24

NEGROIDS

AFRICA

UPPER VOLTA

KURUMBA   REF. 57

PHENOTYPES

OBS.	EXP.	
73	77.0	1, 5, 11, 13, 14
46	39.4	1, 5, 6, 11, 13, 14, 24
3	5.0	1, 5, 6, 11, 24
6	6.5	1, 5, 6, 11, 13, 14,
0	1.6	1, 5, 6, 11, 14, 24
1	0.1	1, 5, 6, 11, 14
16	12.9	1, 5, 11, 13, 14, 15
2	3.3	1, 5, 6, 11, 13, 15, 24
0	0.5	1, 5, 6, 11, 13, 14, 15
0	0.5	1, 11, 13, 15
1	2.1	1, 5, 11, 13, 14, 21
1	0.5	1, 5, 6, 11, 21, 24
1	0.1	1, 5, 6, 11, 14, 21
0	0.2	1, 11, 13, 15, 21
0	0.0	1, 21
TOTAL 150	150.0	

CHI SQUARE= 4.863   D.F. = 4

HAPLOTYPES

FREQ.	S.E.	
0.717	0.026	1, 5, 11, 13, 14
0.183	0.022	1, 5, 6, 11, 13, 24
0.030	0.010	1, 5, 6, 11, 14
0.060	0.014	1, 11, 13, 15
0.010	0.006	1, 21

155

TABLE X-1
TESTED FOR GM 1, 2, 5, 6

PHENOTYPES

POLYNESIANS

OCEANIA

U.S.A.

	TOTAL		1 5	1 2 5	1 2	1	DF	CHI SQ. VALUE
HAWAIIANS HONOLULU, HI.	94	O.	79	14	0	1	1	0
		E.	80.1	12.0	1.5	0.4		

HAPLOTYPES

	1 5	1 2	1	REF.
F.	0.857	0.074	0.069	124
S.E.	0.046	0.019	0.044	

156

TABLE XI-1
TESTED FOR GM 1, 2, 3, 5, 10, 11

PHENOTYPES

OTHER POPULATIONS

AFRICA

		TOTAL	1 5 10 11	1 5 11	1 2 5 10 11	1 2 5 11	1 2	1 3 5 10 11	1 2 3 5 10 11	3 5 10 11	1	CHI SQ. DF	VALUE	REF.
ETHIOPIA														
ADI-ARKAI AND DEBARECH	O.	171	88		4		1	69	1	6	2	2	2.799	48
	E.		92.1		3.8		0.7	60.9	1.5	9.8	2.2			
SUDAN														
BEJA	O.	98	41	6	2	0	1	39	1	3	5	2	2.008	25
	E.		43.1	5.9	1.6	0.4	1.0	34.3	0.9	5.4	5.3			

HAPLOTYPES

OTHER POPULATIONS

AFRICA

		TOTAL	1 5 10 11	1 5 11	1 2 11	3 5 10 11	1	REF.
ETHIOPIA								
ADI-ARKAI AND DEBARECH	F.	171	0.629	0.018		0.240	0.113	48
	S.E.		0.041	0.007		0.023	0.036	
SUDAN								
BEJA	F.	98	0.407	0.105	0.021	0.235	0.234	25
	S.E.		0.047	0.038	0.010	0.030	0.048	

157

TABLE XI-2
TESTED FOR GM 1, 2, 3, 5, 6, 13, 14

OTHER POPULATIONS

AFRICA

SOUTH AFRICA

CAPE COLOUREDS, JOHANNESBURG   REF. 64

PHENOTYPES

OBS.	EXP.	
18	21.0	1, 5, 13, 14
10	7.9	1, 5, 6, 13, 14
2	2.2	1, 5, 6, 14
1	2.9	1, 5, 6, 14
2	1.9	1, 5, 6, 13
6	7.2	1, 13
2	2.2	1
4	2.3	1, 2
2	3.2	1, 2, 5, 13, 14
0	0.8	1, 2, 5, 6, 14
1	0.8	1, 2, 5, 6, 14
2	2.1	1, 2, 13
4	4.2	1, 2, 3, 5, 13, 14
43	35.4	1, 3, 5, 13, 14
9	7.8	1, 3, 5, 6, 13, 14
6	10.3	3, 5, 13, 14
TOTAL 112	112.0	

CHI SQUARE= 7.941   D.F. = 8

HAPLOTYPES

FREQ.	S.E.	
0.231	0.038	1, 5, 13, 14
0.058	0.023	1, 5, 6, 14
0.057	0.022	1, 5, 6, 14
0.150	0.038	1, 13
0.139	0.037	1
0.061	0.016	1, 2
0.304	0.031	3, 5, 13, 14

TABLE XI-3
TESTED FOR GM 1, 2, 3, 5, 6, 11, 13, 14

PHENOTYPES

OTHER POPULATIONS		3 5 11 13 14	1 3 5 11 13 14	1 2 3 5 11 13 14	1 2 13 14	1	1 11 13	1 2 11 13	CHI SQ. DF	VALUE
OCEANIA										
SEYCHELLE ISLANDS	TOTAL									
SEYCHELLE ISLANDERS	157 O.	19	128	1	0	6	2	1		0
	E.	19.0	128.1	0.7	0.5	5.9	2.3	0.5		

HAPLOTYPES

	3 5 14	1 3 5 11 13 14	11 13 14	1	1 2 13	1 11 13	REF.
F.	0.348	0.491	0.065	0.022	0.074		196
S.E.	0.037	0.052	0.037	0.008	0.037		

TABLE XI-4
TESTED FOR GM 1, 2, 3, 5, 6, 13, 14, 21

PHENOTYPES

OTHER POPULATIONS		1 3 5 13 14 21	1 2 3 5 13 14 21	1 3 5 13 14	2 21	1 3 5 13 14	CHI SQ. DF	VALUE
ASIA								
MALAYSIA	TOTAL							
NEGRITOS	48 O.	4	0	24	2	18	1	1.075
	E.	5.3	0.7	20.7	1.3	20.0		

HAPLOTYPES

	1 3 5 13 14	1 2 21	1 3 5 13 14	REF.
F.	0.333	0.021	0.646	169
S.E.	0.048	0.015	0.049	

TABLE XI-4   CONTINUED
TESTED FOR GM 1, 2, 3, 5, 6, 13, 14, 21

OTHER POPULATIONS

AFRICA

ETHIOPIA

SIDAMO   REF. 170

PHENOTYPES

OBS.	EXP.	
28	28.3	1 ; 5, 13, 14
18	17.1	1 ; 5, 6, 13, 14
0	0.0	1 ; 5, 6
2	2.6	1 ; 5, 6, 14
0	0.2	1 ; 5, 6, 13
0	0.5	1 ; 13
5	4.0	1 ; 13, 21
1	0.3	1 ; 2, 13, 21
28	25.9	1 ; 5, 13, 14, 21
3	2.0	1 ; 2, 5, 13, 14, 21
1	0.7	1 ; 5, 6, 21
0	0.1	1 ; 2, 5, 6, 21
8	8.2	1 ; 5, 6, 14, 21
1	0.6	1 ; 2, 5, 6, 14, 21
7	7.8	1 ; 21
0	1.2	1 ; 2, 21
10	10.4	1 ; 3, 5, 13, 14, 21
0	0.8	1 ; 2, 3, 5, 13, 14, 21
16	20.0	1 ; 3, 5, 13, 14
6	6.0	1 ; 3, 5, 6, 13, 14
6	3.5	3 ; 5, 13, 14
TOTAL 140	140.0	

CHI SQUARE= 6.231   D.F.= 8

HAPLOTYPES

FREQ.	S.E.	
0.393	0.034	1 ; 5, 13, 14
0.011	0.011	1 ; 5, 6
0.125	0.022	1 ; 5, 6, 14
0.061	0.023	1 ; 13
0.236	0.025	1 ; 21
0.018	0.008	1 ; 2, 21
0.157	0.022	3 ; 5, 13, 14

TABLE XI-4 CONTINUED
TESTED FOR GM 1, 2, 3, 5, 6, 13, 14, 21

OTHER POPULATIONS

AFRICA

SOUTH AFRICA

!KUBOES-COLOURED   REF. 175

PHENOTYPES

OBS.	EXP.	
34	35.7	1, 5, 13, 14
9	10.7	1, 13
0	1.5	1, 5, 14
13	8.9	1, 5, 13, 14, 21
9	10.9	1, 2, 5, 13, 14, 21
14	12.0	1, 13, 21
18	14.7	1, 2, 13, 21
5	4.5	1, 5, 14, 21
9	5.5	1, 2, 5, 14, 21
0	3.4	1, 21
10	13.4	1, 2, 21
4	1.8	1, 3, 5, 13, 14, 21
2	2.2	1, 2, 3, 5, 13, 14, 21
5	6.6	1, 3, 5, 13, 14
0	0.2	3, 5, 13, 14
TOTAL 132	132.0	

CHI SQUARE=15.075   D.F. = 8

HAPLOTYPES

FREQ.	S.E.	
0.211	0.032	1, 5, 13, 14
0.284	0.031	1, 13
0.107	0.025	1, 5, 14
0.160	0.024	1, 21
0.196	0.025	1, 2, 21
0.042	0.012	3, 5, 13, 14

TABLE XI-5
TESTED FOR GM 1, 2, 3, 5, 6, 13, 14, 17, 21

OTHER POPULATIONS

AFRICA

EGYPT

EGYPTIANS, CAIRO   REF. 176

PHENOTYPES *

OBS.	EXP.	
67	67.1	3, 5, 13, 14
30	25.7	1, 3, 5, 13, 14, 17, 21
2	2.5	1, 17, 21
8	5.8	1, 2, 3, 5, 13, 14, 17, 21
0	1.2	1, 2, 17, 21
69	75.0	1, 3, 5, 13, 14, 17
15	14.4	1, 5, 13, 14, 17, 21
1	3.2	1, 2, 5, 13, 14, 17, 21
24	21.0	1, 5, 13, 14, 17
15	15.2	1, 3, 5, 6, 13, 14, 17
0	2.2	1, 5, 6, 17, 21
1	0.5	1, 2, 5, 6, 17, 21
10	8.5	1, 5, 6, 13, 14, 17
1	0.5	1, 5, 6, 17
0	0.7	1, 5, 6, 14, 17, 21
1	0.2	1, 2, 5, 6, 14, 17, 21
0	0.4	1, 5, 6, 14, 17
TOTAL 244	244.0	

CHI SQUARE= 8.801   D.F. = 8

HAPLOTYPES

FREQ.	S.E.	
0.525	0.023	3, 5, 13, 14
0.100	0.014	1, 17, 21
0.023	0.007	1, 2, 17, 21
0.293	0.021	1, 5, 13, 14, 17
0.045	0.014	1, 5, 6, 17
0.015	0.012	1, 5, 6, 14, 17

* EXCLUDING ONE GM(1, 2, 3, 5, 13, 14, 17) SAMPLE.

TABLE XI-6
TESTED FOR GM 1, 2, 3, 5, 11, 13, 14, 15, 16, 17, 21, 24

PHENOTYPES

OTHER POPULATIONS
ASIA
PHILIPPINES

NEGRITOS

			1 17 21	1 2 17 21	1 3 5 11 13 14 17 21	1 2 3 5 11 13 14 17 21	1 3 5 11 13 14	1 5 11 13 14 17 21	1 2 5 11 13 14 17 21	1 3 5 11 13 14 17	1 5 11 13 14 17	1 5 11 13 14 17 21	1 2 5 11 13 14 15 17 21	1 3 5 11 13 14 15 17	1 5 11 13 14 15 17	DF	CHI SQ. VALUE	REF.
		TOTAL																
AGUSAN MINDANAO	93	O.	2	8	14	27	36	0	0	6	0					3	3.982	84
		E.	1.3	8.7	14.3	24.8	38.1	0.7	1.2	3.8	0.1							
BATAAN LUZON	87	O.	1	5	18	11	47	0	0	5	0					3	3.199	84
		E.	1.6	3.2	17.4	12.8	47.1	0.7	0.5	3.7	0.1							
ZAMBALES LUZON	127	O.	12	12	48	10	40	1	0	2	0	0	1	1	0	3	2.176	84
		E.	13.7	9.2	46.3	13.6	39.1	1.0	0.3	1.7	0.0	0.7	0.2	1.1	0.0			

HAPLOTYPES

OTHER POPULATIONS
ASIA
PHILIPPINES

NEGRITOS

			1 17 21	1 2 17 21	1 3 5 11 13 14	1 5 11 13 14 17	1 5 11 13 14 15 17	REF.
		TOTAL						
AGUSAN MINDANAO	93	F.	0.120	0.208	0.640	0.032		84
		S.E.	0.025	0.031	0.035	0.013		
BATAAN LUZON	87	F.	0.136	0.100	0.736	0.029		84
		S.E.	0.026	0.023	0.033	0.013		
ZAMBALES LUZON	127	F.	0.329	0.097	0.555	0.012	0.008	84
		S.E.	0.030	0.019	0.031	0.007	0.006	

163

TABLE XII-1
TESTED FOR INV 1

ABORIGINES	PHENOTYPES			ALLELE	REF.
	TOTAL	1	−1	1	
OCEANIA					
AUSTRALIA					
BENTINCK ISLAND	33	32	1	F. 0.826 S.E. 0.086	168
CENTRAL REGION	295	118	177	F. 0.225 S.E. 0.018	92
MORNINGTON ISLAND	89	48	41	F. 0.321 S.E. 0.039	168
QUEENSLAND					
AURUNKUN	70	27	43	F. 0.216 S.E. 0.037	159
EDWARD RIVER	81	36	45	F. 0.255 S.E. 0.037	159
MITCHELL RIVER	111	68	43	F. 0.378 S.E. 0.037	159
NORTH	103	54	49	F. 0.310 S.E. 0.036	29
YARRABAH	88	52	36	F. 0.360 S.E. 0.041	159
S. COAST OF GULF OF CARPENTERIA	128	49	79	F. 0.214 S.E. 0.027	168

TABLE XII-2
TESTED FOR INV 2

PHENOTYPES ALLELE

ABORIGINES

OCEANIA

AUSTRALIA

	TOTAL	2	-2		2	REF.
KIMBERLEYS	122	45	77	F.	0.206	121
				S.E.	0.027	
WESTERN DESERT	113	49	64	F.	0.247	121
				S.E.	0.031	

TABLE XII-3
TESTED FOR INV 1, 3

PHENOTYPES ALLELES

ABORIGINES

OCEANIA

AUSTRALIA

	TOTAL		1	1 3	3	DF	CHI SQ. VALUE		1	3	REF.
CENTRAL REGION NO. TERRITORY	84	O.	4	27	53	1	0.055	F.	0.208	0.792	166
		E.	3.6	27.7	52.6			S.E.	0.031	0.031	
NORTH REGION NO. TERRITORY	104	O.	3	24	77	1	0.442	F.	0.144	0.856	166
		E.	2.2	25.7	76.2			S.E.	0.024	0.024	

TABLE XIII-1
TESTED FOR INV 1

PHENOTYPES   ALLELE

AINU

ASIA

JAPAN

	TOTAL	1	—1		1	REF.
HOKKAIDO HIDAKA	407	158	249	F. 0.218 · S.E. 0.015		80
HOKKAIDO	187	58	129	F. 0.169 S.E. 0.020		163
HOKKAIDO	159	49	110	F. 0.168 S.E. 0.022		165

TABLE XIV-1
TESTED FOR INV 1

CAUCASOIDS	PHENOTYPES			ALLELE		REF.
	TOTAL	1	-1	1		
AFRICA						
SOUTH AFRICA						
ASIATIC IND. DURBAN	401	63	338	F. 0.082	S.E. 0.010	64
ASIA						
INDIA						
INDIANS	375	59	316	F. 0.082	S.E. 0.010	187
IRANIS (SAMPLE 1)	54	2	52	F. 0.019	S.E. 0.013	173
IRANIS (SAMPLE 2)	107	1	106	F. 0.005	S.E. 0.005	173
KUMOAN REGION						
BRAHAMINS	102	20	82	F. 0.103	S.E. 0.022	17
DOMS	79	18	61	F. 0.121	S.E. 0.027	17
RAJPUTS	129	50	79	F. 0.217	S.E. 0.027	17
PARSIS	258	17	241	F. 0.034	S.E. 0.008	173
TURKEY						
TURKS	274	39	235	F. 0.074	S.E. 0.011	58

TABLE XIV-1 CONTINUED
TESTED FOR INV 1

	PHENOTYPES			ALLELE	REF.
	TOTAL	1	1 — 1	1	
CAUCASOIDS					
EUROPE					
AUSTRIA					
VIENNA	1334	213	1121	F. 0.083 S.E. 0.005	86
CZECHOSLOVAKIA					
BRNO	876	96	780	F. 0.056 S.E. 0.006	56
CENTRAL BOHEMIA	688	80	608	F. 0.060 S.E. 0.007	146
FINLAND					
ALAND ISLANDS	119	10	109	F. 0.043 S.E. 0.013	174
FINNS INARI	39	2	37	F. 0.026 S.E. 0.018	174
FINNS RISTIINA	100	9	91	F. 0.046 S.E. 0.015	174
GERMANY					
BADEN-WURTTEMBURG	487	79	408	F. 0.085 S.E. 0.009	112
BAYERISCHEN WALD	2000	287	1713	F. 0.075 S.E. 0.004	201
BERLIN	102	9	93	F. 0.045 S.E. 0.015	104
COLOGNE	949	119	830	F. 0.065 S.E. 0.006	58

TABLE XIV-1 CONTINUED
TESTED FOR INV 1

CAUCASOIDS	PHENOTYPES			ALLELE		REF.
	TOTAL	1	-1	1		
EUROPE						
GERMANY						
FREIBURG	1513	236	1277	F. 0.081	S.E. 0.005	58
FREIBURG, MAINZ AND MARBURG	1732	241	1491	F. 0.072	S.E. 0.004	113
HESSEN	2000	268	1732	F. 0.069	S.E. 0.004	199
LINDAU	1300	152	1148	F. 0.060	S.E. 0.005	201
MARBURG	446	71	375	F. 0.083	S.E. 0.009	111
SCHLESWIG-HOLSTEIN	2000	276	1724	F. 0.072	S.E. 0.004	201
SUDLICHEN EIFEL	2250	362	1888	F. 0.084	S.E. 0.004	201
UNTERFRANKEN, OBERFRANKEN	3000	478	2522	F. 0.083	S.E. 0.004	201
WURZBURG	2000	293	1707	F. 0.076	S.E. 0.004	200
GREECE						
ACHAIA, N. W. PELOPONNESUS	150	21	129	F. 0.073	S.E. 0.015	2
GHAVRIA ARTA PREFECTURE	344	95	249	F. 0.149	S.E. 0.014	32

TABLE XIV-1 CONTINUED
TESTED FOR INV 1

	PHENOTYPES			ALLELE	REF.
	TOTAL	1	−1	1	
CAUCASOIDS					
EUROPE					
GREECE					
GREEKS	256	32	224	F. 0.065 S.E. 0.011	2
GREEKS	218	32	186	F. 0.076 S.E. 0.013	193
KALOVATOS ARTA PREFECTURE	317	75	242	F. 0.126 S.E. 0.014	32
HUNGARY					
BUDAPEST	5000	605	4395	F. 0.062 S.E. 0.002	107
BUDAPEST	184	26	158	F. 0.073 S.E. 0.014	145
CIGAND	151	29	122	F. 0.101 S.E. 0.018	192
KARCSA	120	14	106	F. 0.060 S.E. 0.016	192
KISROZVAGY/ NAGYROZVAGY	145	19	126	F. 0.068 S.E. 0.015	192
OTHER ORIGIN	128	19	109	F. 0.077 S.E. 0.017	192
ICELAND					
DALASYSLA	193	34	159	F. 0.092 S.E. 0.015	95

TABLE XIV-1 CONTINUED
TESTED FOR INV 1

PHENOTYPES ALLELE

CAUCASOIDS	TOTAL	1	1-1		1	REF.
EUROPE						
IRELAND						
IRISH	294	43	251	F. S. E.	0.076 0.011	96
ITALY						
FERRARA	86	14	72	F. S. E.	0.085 0.022	100
MOUNTAIN SARDINIA	203	44	159	F. S. E.	0.115 0.016	100
NORTH SARDINIA	444	82	362	F. S. E.	0.097 0.010	100
NORTHEAST SARDINIA	198	24	174	F. S. E.	0.063 0.012	100
SOUTH SARDINIA	182	43	139	F. S. E.	0.126 0.018	100
SOUTHEAST SARDINIA	191	33	158	F. S. E.	0.090 0.015	100
NORWAY						
NORWEGIANS	87	12	75	F. S. E.	0.072 0.020	35
POLAND						
LOWER SILESIA	1051	142	909	F. S. E.	0.070 0.006	147

TABLE XIV-1 CONTINUED TESTED FOR INV 1

CAUCASOIDS	PHENOTYPES			ALLELE		REF.
	TOTAL	1	1 — 1	1		
EUROPE						
SWITZERLAND						
SWISS	98	15	83	F. 0.080	S.E. 0.020	178
U.S.S.R.						
MARIS KOZMODEMYANSK	110	3	107	F. 0.014	S.E. 0.008	174
MARIS VOLZHSK	101	9	92	F. 0.046	S.E. 0.015	174
MARIS ZVENIGOVO	103	4	99	F. 0.020	S.E. 0.010	174
YUGOSLAVIA						
DUBROVNIK, STON AND METKOVIK	121	16	105	F. 0.068	S.E. 0.017	30
GYPSIES OF SKOPJE	36	3	33	F. 0.043	S.E. 0.024	30
RIJEKA	134	16	118	F. 0.062	S.E. 0.015	30
SPLIT, BIOGRAD AND ZADAR	197	18	179	F. 0.047	S.E. 0.011	30
YUGOSLAVIANS	505	54	451	F. 0.055	S.E. 0.007	30

TABLE XIV-1 CONTINUED
TESTED FOR INV 1

		PHENOTYPES			ALLELE		
		TOTAL	1	-1		1	REF.
CAUCASOIDS							
MIDDLE EAST							
IRAN							
CENTRAL AND SOUTH		223	44	179	F. S.E.	0.104 0.015	4
EAST		168	45	123	F. S.E.	0.144 0.020	4
NORTH		167	48	119	F. S.E.	0.156 0.021	4
NORTHWEST		227	56	171	F. S.E.	0.132 0.016	4
TEHERAN		354	98	256	F. S.E.	0.150 0.014	4
WEST		286	64	222	F. S.E.	0.119 0.014	4
N. AMERICA							
CUBA							
SANTIAGO DE CUBA		182	93	89	F. S.E.	0.301 0.026	52
OCEANIA							
AUSTRALIA							
MIXED, MAINLY BRITISH	460	362	98		F. S.E.	0.538 0.021	189

TABLE XIV-2
TESTED FOR INV 2

		PHENOTYPES		ALLELE	
	TOTAL	2	-2	2	REF.
CAUCASOIDS					
EUROPE					
CZECHOSLOVAKIA					
PRAGUE	190	23	167	F. 0.062 S.E. 0.013	122
PRAGUE	445	39	406	F. 0.045 S.E. 0.007	49
PRAGUE	96	15	81	F. 0.081 S.E. 0.020	50
FINLAND					
HELSINKI	162	18	144	F. 0.057 S.E. 0.013	122
FRANCE					
SEINE-MARITIME	324	60	264	F. 0.097 S.E. 0.012	116
SEINE-MARITIME	402	78	324	F. 0.102 S.E. 0.011	117
GERMANY					
LEIPZIG	164	16	148	F. 0.050 S.E. 0.012	60
LEIPZIG	2220	271	1949	F. 0.063 S.E. 0.004	51
MUNICH	148	17	131	F. 0.059 S.E. 0.014	122

TABLE XIV-2 CONTINUED
TESTED FOR INV 2

| | PHENOTYPES | | | ALLELE | |
	TOTAL	2	-2	2	REF.
CAUCASOIDS					
EUROPE					
GREECE					
ATHENS	297	51	246	F. 0.090 S.E. 0.012	122
NETHERLANDS					
DUTCH	354	57	297	F. 0.084 S.E. 0.011	122
YUGOSLAVIA					
LJUBLJANA	157	23	134	F. 0.076 S.E. 0.015	122
MIDDLE EAST					
IRAN					
IRANIANS	297	34	263	F. 0.059 S.E. 0.010	119

TABLE XIV-3
TESTED FOR INV 1,2

		PHENOTYPES				ALLELES			REF.
		TOTAL	1	1·2	−1·−2	1	1·2	−1·−2	
CAUCASOIDS									
EUROPE									
DENMARK									
DANES	F.	105		19	86		0.095	0.905	131
	S.E.						0.021	0.021	
FRANCE									
NORMANDY	F.	331	2	65	264	0.003	0.104	0.893	127
	S.E.					0.002	0.012	0.012	
GERMANY									
FREIBURG	F.	428	1	49	378	0.001	0.059	0.940	110
	S.E.					0.001	0.008	0.008	
GERMANS	F.	782		99	683		0.065	0.935	109
	S.E.						0.006	0.006	
RHEINLAND-PFALZ	F.	386		41	345		0.055	0.945	125
	S.E.						0.008	0.008	
HUNGARY									
BUDAPEST	F.	63		5	58		0.041	0.959	130
	S.E.						0.018	0.018	
HEVES	F.	105	2	9	94	0.010	0.044	0.946	130
	S.E.					0.007	0.014	0.016	
IRAD	F.	210		17	193		0.041	0.959	130
	S.E.						0.010	0.010	
ICELAND									
ICELANDERS	F.	69	1	18	50	0.008	0.140	0.851	98
	S.E.					0.008	0.031	0.032	

TABLE XIV-3 CONTINUED
TESTED FOR INV 1,2

CAUCASOIDS

EUROPE

		PHENOTYPES				ALLELES			REF.
	TOTAL	1	1-2	-1-2		1	1-2	-1-2	
NETHERLANDS									
DUTCH	798	1	142	655	F.	0.001	0.093	0.906	31
					S.E.	0.001	0.007	0.007	
POLAND									
KRACOW REGION	600	1	63	536	F.	0.001	0.054	0.945	151
					S.E.	0.001	0.007	0.007	
SWITZERLAND									
SWISS	600	4	106	490	F.	0.004	0.093	0.904	73
					S.E.	0.002	0.009	0.009	
UNITED KINGDOM									
BRITISH	500	8	80	412	F.	0.009	0.083	0.908	13
					S.E.	0.003	0.009	0.009	
YUGOSLAVIA									
BISTARC	148	1	11	136	F.	0.004	0.038	0.959	132
					S.E.	0.004	0.011	0.012	
BLJECEVA	184		14	170	F.		0.039	0.961	132
					S.E.		0.010	0.010	
KOCEVICI	196		18	178	F.		0.047	0.953	132
					S.E.		0.011	0.011	
OCEVLGE- VLAHINJE	149		9	140	F.		0.031	0.969	132
					S.E.		0.010	0.010	

MIDDLE EAST

IRAN

	TOTAL	1	1-2	-1-2		1	1-2	-1-2	REF.
KURDISTANI	167		23	144	F.		0.071	0.929	8
					S.E.		0.014	0.014	

177

TABLE XIV-4
TESTED FOR INV 1, 3

PHENOTYPES   ALLELES

CAUCASOIDS

N. AMERICA

U.S.A.

	TOTAL	1	1 3	3	DF	CHI SQ. VALUE		1	3	REF.
CLAXTON, GA.	295	O.	1	39	255	1	0.146	F.	0.069	0.931	10
		E.	1.4	38.2	255.4			S.E.	0.010	0.010	

TABLE XIV-5
TESTED FOR INV 2

PHENOTYPES   ALLELE

CAUCASOIDS-ARABS

AFRICA

ALGERIA

	TOTAL	2	2 -2	-2		2	REF.
NOMADS	68	23	45		F.	0.187	117
					S.E.	0.035	
REGUIBAT TINDOUF	199	121	78		F.	0.374	118
					S.E.	0.028	
REGUIBAT TINDOUF	324	142	182		F.	0.251	123
					S.E.	0.018	
TADJAKANT TINDOUF	57	33	24		F.	0.351	118
					S.E.	0.050	
TADJAKANT TINDOUF	58	22	36		F.	0.212	123
					S.E.	0.040	

TABLE XIV-6
TESTED FOR INV 1

PHENOTYPES   ALLELE

CAUCASOIDS-JEWS

N. AMERICA

U.S.A.

	TOTAL	1 -1		1	REF.
ASHKENAZIC JEWS	248	18	230	F. 0.037	171
				S.E. 0.009	

TABLE XIV-7
TESTED FOR INV 1, 2

PHENOTYPES   ALLELES

CAUCASOIDS-JEWS

MIDDLE EAST

ISRAEL

	TOTAL	1 -1	2 -2		1 -1	2 -2	REF.
KURDISH JEWS	88	1	87	F.	0.006	0.994	41
				S.E.	0.006	0.006	
YEMENITE JEWS	75	14	61	F.	0.098	0.902	41
				S.E.	0.025	0.025	

TABLE XV-1
TESTED FOR INV 1

KHOISAN-KHOIKHOI

AFRICA

S.W. AFRICA

| | | PHENOTYPES | | ALLELE | |
	TOTAL	1	−1	1	REF.
KEETMANSHOOP	150	90	60	F. 0.368 S.E. 0.032	175
SESFONTEIN	42	25	17	F. 0.364 S.E. 0.060	175
TOPNAAR KUISEB VALLEY	57	17	40	F. 0.162 S.E. 0.036	63

TABLE XV-1 CONTINUED
TESTED FOR INV 1

KHOISAN-SAN

AFRICA

BOTSWANA

		PHENOTYPES			ALLELE		
	TOTAL	1	−1			1	REF.
CENTRAL-SOUTH KALAHARI DES	112	62	50		F. S. E.	0.332 0.035	62
KAUKAU GHANZI	263	150	113		F. S. E.	0.345 0.023	175
!KUNG /AI/AI	62	35	27		F. S. E.	0.340 0.048	175
!KUNG /DU/DA	100	60	40		F. S. E.	0.368 0.039	175
!KUNG DOBE	394	253	141		F. S. E.	0.402 0.020	175
!KUNG NGAMI	156	97	59		F. S. E.	0.385 0.032	175
!KUNG NORTHERN	103	62	41		F. S. E.	0.369 0.038	175
MAINLY SOUTHERN	72	37	35		F. S. E.	0.303 0.042	64
NARON GHANZI	140	82	58		F. S. E.	0.356 0.032	175

TABLE XVI-1
TESTED FOR INV 1

LAPPS

EUROPE

FINLAND

PHENOTYPES   ALLELE

	TOTAL	1	-1		1	REF.
NELLIM SKOLT	130	36	94	F.	0.150	174
				S.E.	0.023	

TABLE XVI-2
TESTED FOR INV 1, 3

PHENOTYPES   ALLELES

LAPPS

EUROPE

FINLAND

	TOTAL		1	1 3	3	DF	CHI SQ. VALUE		1	3	REF.
FISHER	142	O.	1	47	94	1	3.598	F.	0.173	0.827	174
		E.	4.2	40.5	97.2			S.E.	0.022	0.022	
MOUNTAIN	125	O.	4	37	84	1	0.001	F.	0.180	0.820	174
		E.	4.1	36.9	84.1			S.E.	0.024	0.024	
SEVETTIJARVI SKOLT	206	O.	8	74	124	1	0.558	F.	0.218	0.782	174
		E.	9.8	70.3	125.8			S.E.	0.020	0.020	

TABLE XVII-1
TESTED FOR INV 1

MELANESIANS	PHENOTYPES			ALLELE	REF.
	TOTAL	1	1-1	1	
OCEANIA					
FIJI					
LAU ISLANDS	74	11	63	F. 0.077 S.E. 0.022	139
VITI LEVU	96	29	67	F. 0.165 S.E. 0.028	139
SOLOMON IS.					
BOUGAINVILLE					
ALL MN SPEAKERS	351	208	143	F. 0.362 S.E. 0.021	33
ALL NAN SPEAKERS	1803	1396	407	F. 0.525 S.E. 0.010	33
ARAWA VILLAGE MN	108	59	49	F. 0.326 S.E. 0.036	33
ROROVANA VILLAGE MN	243	149	94	F. 0.378 S.E. 0.025	33
ATAMO VILLAGE NAN	124	109	15	F. 0.652 S.E. 0.042	33
BAIRIMA VILLAGE NAN	59	43	16	F. 0.479 S.E. 0.056	33
BOIRA VILLAGE NAN	84	55	29	F. 0.412 S.E. 0.044	33
KARNAVITU VILLAGE NAN	133	97	36	F. 0.480 S.E. 0.037	33

TABLE XVII-1 CONTINUED
TESTED FOR INV 1

MELANESIANS

OCEANIA

SOLOMON IS.

| | | PHENOTYPES | | | ALLELE | |
| | | | | | | |
	TOTAL	1	-1		1	REF.
BOUGAINVILLE						
KOPANI VILLAGE	NAN 190	165	25	F.	0.637	33
				S.E.	0.034	
KOPIKIRI VILLAGE	NAN 70	64	6	F.	0.707	33
				S.E.	0.057	
KORPEI VILLAGE	NAN 181	119	62	F.	0.415	33
				S.E.	0.030	
MORONEI VILLAGE	NAN 112	69	43	F.	0.380	33
				S.E.	0.037	
NASIWOIWA VILLAGE	NAN 128	116	12	F.	0.694	33
				S.E.	0.042	
NUPATORO VILLAGE	NAN 99	96	3	F.	0.826	33
				S.E.	0.049	
OKOWAPAIPA VILLAGE	NAN 94	87	7	F.	0.727	33
				S.E.	0.050	
OLD SIUAI VILLAGE	NAN 25	18	7	F.	0.471	33
				S.E.	0.085	
POMAUA VILLAGE	NAN 116	85	31	F.	0.483	33
				S.E.	0.040	
RUMBA VILLAGE	NAN 148	97	51	F.	0.413	33
				S.E.	0.033	
SIERONJI VILLAGE	NAN 62	42	20	F.	0.432	33
				S.E.	0.052	

TABLE XVII-1 CONTINUED
TESTED FOR INV 1

		PHENOTYPES			ALLELE	
	TOTAL	1	1-1		1	REF.

MELANESIANS

OCEANIA

SOLOMON IS.

BOUGAINVILLE

TURUNGUM VILLAGE NAN	88	63	25	F. S.E.	0.467 0.045	33
URUTO VILLAGE NAN	90	71	19	F. S.E.	0.541 0.047	33
AITA NAN	307	287	20	F. S.E.	0.745 0.028	167
NAGOVISI NAN	386	201	185	F. S.E.	0.308 0.018	167
NASIOI RUMBA VILLAGE NAN	161	98	63	F. S.E.	0.374 0.031	167

NEW BRITAIN

| KILENGE | 75 | 17 | 58 | F.
S.E. | 0.121
0.027 | 139 |

NEW GUINEA

AUSTRONESIAN SPEAKERS	948	128	820	F. S.E.	0.070 0.006	40
NAN SPEAKERS	721	156	565	F. S.E.	0.115 0.009	40
ALL MN SPEAKERS	537	64	473	F. S.E.	0.061 0.007	139
ALL NAN SPEAKERS	543	47	496	F. S.E.	0.044 0.006	139

185

TABLE XVII-1 CONTINUED
TESTED FOR INV 1

MELANESIANS

OCEANIA

PAP. N. GUINEA		PHENOTYPES			ALLELE	REF.
		TOTAL	1 1	1 -1	1	

NEW GUINEA

		TOTAL	1 1	1 -1	1	REF.
AWAN VILLAGE	MN	102	8	94	F. 0.040 S.E. 0.014	139
INTOAP VILLAGE	MN	84	11	73	F. 0.068 S.E. 0.020	139
ITSINGATS VILLAGE	MN	66	12	54	F. 0.095 S.E. 0.026	139
PUGUAP VILLAGE	MN	90	6	84	F. 0.034 S.E. 0.014	139
SINGAS VILLAGE	MN	87	13	74	F. 0.078 S.E. 0.021	139
YANUF VILLAGE	MN	41	4	37	F. 0.050 S.E. 0.024	139
YATSING VILLAGE	MN	67	10	57	F. 0.078 S.E. 0.024	139
ASMAT AGATS VILLAGE	NAN	178	26	152	F. 0.076 S.E. 0.014	139
AWIN FLY RIVER	NAN	133	9	124	F. 0.034 S.E. 0.011	139
YANGGAN FLY RIVER	NAN	91	8	83	F. 0.045 S.E. 0.016	139
WAFFA MARKHAM VALL.	NAN	141	4	137	F. 0.014 S.E. 0.007	139

TABLE XVII-1 CONTINUED
TESTED FOR INV 1

MELANESIANS

OCEANIA

PAP. N. GUINEA

	PHENOTYPES			ALLELE		
	TOTAL	1	1-1		1	REF.
NEW GUINEA						
NORTH FORE NAN E. HIGHLANDS	43	0	43	F. S.E.	0.000 0.000	168
SOUTH FORE NAN E. HIGHLANDS	51	2	49	F. S.E.	0.020 0.014	168
USURUFA NAN E. HIGHLANDS	97	5	92	F. S.E.	0.026 0.012	168
HULI S. HIGHLANDS	149	2	147	F. S.E.	0.007 0.005	168
ONABASULA S. HIGHLANDS	231	10	221	F. S.E.	0.022 0.007	168
BAIMI W. DISTRICT	245	4	241	F. S.E.	0.008 0.004	168
OLSOBIP W. DISTRICT	92	4	88	F. S.E.	0.022 0.011	168
SOLOMON IS.						
MALAITA						
KWAIO MN	451	177	274	F. S.E.	0.221 0.015	167

TABLE XVII-2
TESTED FOR INV 1,2

		PHENOTYPES			ALLELES		
MELANESIANS		1-1	2-2		1	2	
OCEANIA	TOTAL	1-2					REF.
PAP. N. GUINEA							
NEW BRITAIN							
BAINING NAN GAULIM VILLAGE	42	16	26	F.	0.213	0.787	18
				S.E.	0.048	0.048	
TOLAI MN							
KOULON VILLAGE	44	6	38	F.	0.071	0.929	18
				S.E.	0.028	0.028	
KURAIP VILLAGE	35	3	32	F.	0.044	0.956	18
				S.E.	0.025	0.025	
NORDUP VILLAGE	38	16	22	F.	0.239	0.761	18
				S.E.	0.053	0.053	
RAKUNAI VILLAGE	16	4	12	F.	0.134	0.866	18
				S.E.	0.063	0.063	
NEW GUINEA							
ENGA NAN LAIAGAM VILL.	185	10	175	F.	0.027	0.973	18
				S.E.	0.009	0.009	
GOGODARA NAN BALIMO VILLAGE	99	15	84	F.	0.079	0.921	18
				S.E.	0.020	0.020	
KUMAN NAN MINJ VILLAGE	101	1	100	F.	0.005	0.995	18
				S.E.	0.005	0.005	
MOTU MN POREBADA VILL.	38	20	18	F.	0.312	0.688	18
				S.E.	0.059	0.059	

TABLE XVII-3
TESTED FOR INV 1,3

MELANESIANS

OCEANIA

SOLOMON IS.

MALAITA

		PHENOTYPES			CHI SQ.		ALLELES		
	TOTAL	1	1 3	3	DF	VALUE	1	3	REF.
BAEGU MN	147	O. 7	52	88			F. 0.224	0.776	
		E. 7.4	51.2	88.4	1	0.037	S.E. 0.024	0.024	167
LAU MN	143	O. 4	60	79			F. 0.238	0.762	
		E. 8.1	51.8	83.1	1	3.551	S.E. 0.025	0.025	167

TABLE XVIII-1
TESTED FOR INV 1

MICRONESIANS

OCEANIA

CAROLINE ISLANDS

		PHENOTYPES		ALLELE		
	TOTAL	1	1 -1	-1	1	REF.
KUSAIEANS	254	70	184		F. 0.149	
					S.E. 0.016	172
MOKILESE	207	86	121		F. 0.235	
					S.E. 0.022	172
PINGELAPESE	409	181	228		F. 0.253	
					S.E. 0.016	172
PONAPEANS	190	54	136		F. 0.154	
					S.E. 0.019	172
WEST TRUK	48	17	31		F. 0.196	
					S.E. 0.043	139

189

TABLE XIX-1
TESTED FOR INV 1

| | PHENOTYPES | | | ALLELE | |
	TOTAL	1	−1	1	REF.
MONGOLOIDS					
ASIA					
HONG KONG					
CHINESE	203	105	98	F. 0.305 S.E. 0.025	141
INDIA					
THARUS KUMOAN REGION	152	75	77	F. 0.288 S.E. 0.028	17
JAPAN					
JAPANESE HOKKAIDO	87	49	38	F. 0.339 S.E. 0.040	165
JAPANESE	94	54	40	F. 0.348 S.E. 0.039	70
KAWASAKA-SHI	258	125	133	F. 0.282 S.E. 0.022	182
KUMAMOTO	140	67	73	F. 0.278 S.E. 0.029	183
MIE PREFECTURE	566	287	279	F. 0.298 S.E. 0.015	144
NIIGATA PREFECTURE	201	100	101	F. 0.291 S.E. 0.025	144

190

TABLE XIX-1   CONTINUED
TESTED FOR INV 1

PHENOTYPES   ALLELE

MONGOLIODS

	TOTAL	1	1 -1		1	REF.
ASIA						
JAPAN						
YAMAGATA PREFECTURE	200	114	86	F. 0.344 S.E. 0.027		144
KOREA						
KOREANS	115	57	58	F. 0.290 S.E. 0.033		5
KOREANS	211	109	102	F. 0.305 S.E. 0.025		143
MALAYSIA						
ABORIGINES	68	23	45	F. 0.187 S.E. 0.035		169
SEMAI	175	93	82	F. 0.315 S.E. 0.028		169
MIYAKO						
RYUKYUANS	200	76	124	F. 0.213 S.E. 0.022		90
N. VIETNAM						
VIETNAMESE KINH	153	61	92	F. 0.225 S.E. 0.026		54

191

TABLE XIX-1 CONTINUED
TESTED FOR INV 1

	PHENOTYPES			ALLELE		REF.
	TOTAL	1	-1	1		

MONGOLOIDS

ASIA

OKINAWA

	TOTAL	1	-1			REF.
HANADA CITY	200	97	103	F. 0.282	S.E. 0.025	144
RYUKYUANS HANADA CITY	200	90	110	F. 0.258	S.E. 0.024	90

REP OF CHINA

CHINESE

	TOTAL	1	-1			REF.
NORTH	161	106	55	F. 0.416	S.E. 0.032	90
NORTH	174	103	71	F. 0.361	S.E. 0.029	142
SOUTH	143	81	62	F. 0.342	S.E. 0.031	90
SOUTH	331	170	161	F. 0.303	S.E. 0.020	142

TAIWAN

ABORIGINES

	TOTAL	1	-1			REF.
AMI	152	61	91	F. 0.226	S.E. 0.026	139
AMI	225	104	121	F. 0.267	S.E. 0.023	90
ATAYAL	128	37	91	F. 0.157	S.E. 0.024	139

TABLE XIX-1 CONTINUED
TESTED FOR INV 1

	PHENOTYPES			ALLELE	
MONGOLOIDS	TOTAL	1	1 -1	1	REF.
ASIA					
TAIWAN					
ABORIGINES					
ATAYAL	263	88	175	F. 0.184 S.E. 0.018	90
ATAYAL	154	56	98	F. 0.202 S.E. 0.024	79
BUNUN	36	12	24	F. 0.184 S.E. 0.048	139
BUNUN	103	41	62	F. 0.224 S.E. 0.031	90
BUNUN	104	35	69	F. 0.185 S.E. 0.028	79
PAIWAN	48	15	33	F. 0.171 S.E. 0.040	139
PAIWAN	178	66	112	F. 0.207 S.E. 0.023	90
PAIWAN	210	79	131	F. 0.210 S.E. 0.021	79
CHINESE	200	113	87	F. 0.340 S.E. 0.027	90
CHINESE	214	110	104	F. 0.303 S.E. 0.025	142
TAIWANESE TAICHUNG CITY	286	147	139	F. 0.303 S.E. 0.021	83

TABLE XIX-1 CONTINUED
TESTED FOR INV 1

	PHENOTYPES			ALLELE		
	TOTAL	1	1-1		1	REF.
MONGOLOIDS						
ASIA						
THAILAND						
HILL TRIBES						
KAREN	39	8	31	F.	0.108	139
				S.E.	0.036	
LAHU	71	47	24	F.	0.419	139
				S.E.	0.048	
LISU	26	17	9	F.	0.412	139
				S.E.	0.079	
MEO	110	80	30	F.	0.478	139
				S.E.	0.041	
THAIS						
CENTRAL	128	20	108	F.	0.081	139
				S.E.	0.017	
CENTRAL	887	299	588	F.	0.186	187
				S.E.	0.010	
NORTH	101	32	69	F.	0.173	187
				S.E.	0.028	
NORTH	150	54	96	F.	0.200	139
				S.E.	0.024	
NORTHEAST	197	50	147	F.	0.136	139
				S.E.	0.018	
SOUTH	155	45	110	F.	0.158	139
				S.E.	0.022	

TABLE XIX-1 CONTINUED
TESTED FOR INV 1

	PHENOTYPES			ALLELE	REF.
	TOTAL	1	-1	1	
MONGOLOIDS					
ASIA					
THAILAND					
THAIS	162	92	70	F. 0.343 S.E. 0.030	99
THAIS	479	157	322	F. 0.180 S.E. 0.013	160
THAIS	228	77	151	F. 0.186 S.E. 0.019	161
THAIS	200	59	141	F. 0.160 S.E. 0.019	72
VIETNAM					
VIETNAMESE	414	188	226	F. 0.261 S.E. 0.017	185
C. AMERICA					
MEXICO					
CHOLS INDIANS	142	68	74	F. 0.278 S.E. 0.029	164
CORAS INDIANS	98	34	64	F. 0.192 S.E. 0.030	164
HAUSTECOS INDIANS	173	103	70	F. 0.364 S.E. 0.029	164
MAZATECOS INDIANS	122	71	51	F. 0.353 S.E. 0.035	164
ZAPATECOS INDIANS	98	57	41	F. 0.353 S.E. 0.039	164

TABLE XIX-1 CONTINUED
TESTED FOR INV 1

	PHENOTYPES			ALLELE		
MONGOLOIDS	TOTAL	1	1—1		1	REF.
N. AMERICA						
CANADA						
ESKIMOS IGLOOLIK	365	170	195	F. 0.269 / S.E. 0.018		86
OJIBWA IND. PINKANGIKUM	102	50	52	F. 0.286 / S.E. 0.035		179
OJIBWA IND. WIKWEMIKONG	117	69	48	F. 0.359 / S.E. 0.035		179
GREENLAND						
ESKIMOS AUGPILAGTOK IS. UPERNAVIK DIST.	144	37	107	F. 0.138 / S.E. 0.021		174
S. AMERICA						
BRAZIL						
CAYAPO IND.						
KUBEN-KRAN-KEGN	134	82	52	F. 0.377 / S.E. 0.034		138
MEKRANOTI	93	55	38	F. 0.361 / S.E. 0.040		138
TXUKAHAMAE	154	115	39	F. 0.497 / S.E. 0.035		138
XIKRIN	59	38	21	F. 0.403 / S.E. 0.052		138
AWEIKOMA IND. SANTA CATARINA	27	11	16	F. 0.230 / S.E. 0.061		137

TABLE XIX-1 CONTINUED
TESTED FOR INV 1

MONGOLOIDS

		PHENOTYPES		ALLELE	
	TOTAL	1	-1	1	REF.
S. AMERICA					
BRAZIL					
CAINGANG IND. SANTA CATARINA	52	34	18	F. 0.412 S.E. 0.056	137
CAINGANG MEST. SANTA CATARINA	106	51	55	F. 0.280 S.E. 0.034	137
GUARINI IND. SANTA CATARINA	31	16	15	F. 0.304 S.E. 0.065	137
XAVANTE IND. SAO MARCOS	248	150	98	F. 0.371 S.E. 0.025	150
XAVANTE IND. SIMOES LOPES	143	123	20	F. 0.626 S.E. 0.039	150
PARAGUAY					
NORTHWEST					
AYORE INDIANS	71	42	29	F. 0.361 S.E. 0.046	14
CHEROTI INDIANS	28	5	23	F. 0.094 S.E. 0.040	14
CHULUPI INDIANS	121	43	78	F. 0.197 S.E. 0.027	14
GUARAYU INDIANS	14	11	3	F. 0.537 S.E. 0.118	14
LENGUA INDIANS	45	39	6	F. 0.635 S.E. 0.069	14

TABLE XIX-1 CONTINUED
TESTED FOR INV 1

MONGOLOIDS

S. AMERICA

PARAGUAY

		PHENOTYPES		ALLELE	REF.
	TOTAL	1	−1	1	
NORTHWEST					
SANAPANA INDIANS	97	81	16	F. 0.594 S.E. 0.046	14
TAPIETE INDIANS	19	17	2	F. 0.676 S.E. 0.109	14
TOBA INDIANS	42	39	3	F. 0.733 S.E. 0.074	14
SOUTHWEST					
GUAYAKI INDIANS	61	16	45	F. 0.141 S.E. 0.033	14
SURINAM					
TRIO INDIANS	376	242	134	F. 0.403 S.E. 0.021	37
WAJANA INDIANS	192	113	79	F. 0.359 S.E. 0.028	37
VENEZUELA					
PARAUJANO INDIANS	112	65	47	F. 0.352 S.E. 0.036	34
PIAROA INDIANS	68	64	4	F. 0.757 S.E. 0.059	34
WAICA INDIANS	102	67	35	F. 0.414 S.E. 0.040	34

TABLE XIX-2
TESTED FOR INV 2

MONGOLOIDS	PHENOTYPES			ALLELE		
	TOTAL	2	-2		2	REF.
ASIA						
JAPAN						
JAPANESE	270	129	141	F.	0.277	117
				S.E.	0.021	
TOKYO	109	56	53	F.	0.303	115
				S.E.	0.034	
MACAO						
CHINESE	507	283	224	F.	0.335	123
				S.E.	0.017	

TABLE XIX-3
TESTED FOR INV 1,2

		PHENOTYPES			ALLELES				REF.
MONGOLOIDS	TOTAL	1	1/2	1/-2		1	1/2	1/-2	
C. AMERICA									
MEXICO									
CHIPAS INDIANS AGUACATENANGO	137	3	85	49	F.	0.018	0.384	0.598	26
					S.E.	0.010	0.034	0.034	
OCEANIA									
U.S.A.									
FILIPINOS HONOLULU, HI.	126	6	67	53	F.	0.036	0.316	0.649	124
					S.E.	0.014	0.032	0.034	
N. AMERICA									
GREENLAND									
ESKIMOS ANGMAGSSALIK	65	4	20	41	F.	0.038	0.168	0.794	98
					S.E.	0.019	0.034	0.038	
ESKIMOS WEST COAST	47	2	12	33	F.	0.025	0.137	0.838	98
					S.E.	0.017	0.037	0.040	
POLAR ESKIMOS THULE	29	1	10	18	F.	0.022	0.191	0.788	98
					S.E.	0.021	0.055	0.057	
ESKIMOS JULIANEHAB	54		21	33	F.		0.218	0.782	98
					S.E.		0.042	0.042	
S. AMERICA									
BOLIVIA									
CHIPAYA INDIANS	77		64	13	F.		0.589	0.411	105
					S.E.		0.052	0.052	

TABLE XIX-3 CONTINUED
TESTED FOR INV 1,2

PHENOTYPES   ALLELES

MONGOLOIDS

S. AMERICA

FRENCH GUIANA	TOTAL	1 -1 2 -2			1 2	-1 -2	REF.
EMERILLON INDIANS	38	9	29	F.	0.126	0.874	21
				S.E.	0.039	0.039	
OYAMPI INDIANS OYAPOK	99	84	15	F.	0.611	0.389	21
				S.E.	0.046	0.046	
WAYANA INDIANS MARONI	165	95	70	F.	0.349	0.651	21
				S.E.	0.030	0.030	

TABLE XIX-4
TESTED FOR INV 1,3

PHENOTYPES   ALLELES

MONGOLOIDS

ASIA

JAPAN

	TOTAL		1 3	3	CHI SQ. DF VALUE		1 3	REF.
JAPANESE OSAKA	748	O.	81	291	376	1 4.623	F. 0.303 0.697	157
		E.	68.6	315.8	363.6		S.E. 0.012 0.012	

TABLE XX-1
TESTED FOR INV 1

	PHENOTYPES			ALLELE		
	TOTAL	1	1-1		1	REF.
NEGROIDS						
AFRICA						
ANGOLA						
MIXED TRIBES	111	64	47	F.	0.349	64
				S.E.	0.036	
BOTSWANA						
BECHUANA	155	85	70	F.	0.328	64
				S.E.	0.030	
NGALAGADI	48	32	16	F.	0.423	62
				S.E.	0.059	
GAMBIA						
KENEBA	822	545	277	F.	0.419	177
				S.E.	0.014	
MANDUAR	307	187	120	F.	0.375	177
				S.E.	0.022	
KENYA						
CENTRAL NYANZA DISTRICT	366	230	136	F.	0.390	53
				S.E.	0.021	
LESOTHO						
BASUTU	149	78	71	F.	0.310	64
				S.E.	0.030	
MALAWI						
MIXED TRIBES	153	109	44	F.	0.464	64
				S.E.	0.034	

TABLE XX-1 CONTINUED
TESTED FOR INV 1

NEGROIDS	PHENOTYPES			ALLELE		REF.
	TOTAL	1	−1	1		
AFRICA						
MOZAMBIQUE						
BITONGA	233	154	79	F. 0.418	S.E. 0.027	85
CHANGANE	122	84	38	F. 0.442	S.E. 0.038	85
CHOPE	29	19	10	F. 0.413	S.E. 0.075	85
NYAMBAAN	119	66	53	F. 0.333	S.E. 0.034	64
RONGA	45	33	12	F. 0.484	S.E. 0.064	85
SENA	85	50	35	F. 0.358	S.E. 0.042	85
SHANGAAN TONGA	153	95	58	F. 0.384	S.E. 0.032	64
SOUTH AFRICA						
BACA	137	80	57	F. 0.355	S.E. 0.033	64
HLUBI	147	104	43	F. 0.459	S.E. 0.035	64
NDEBELE TRANSVAAL	129	75	54	F. 0.353	S.E. 0.034	64
PEDI	147	43	104	F. 0.159	S.E. 0.022	64

203

TABLE XX-1 CONTINUED
TESTED FOR INV 1

| | PHENOTYPES | | | ALLELE | |
	TOTAL	1	−1	1	REF.
NEGROIDS					
AFRICA					
SOUTH AFRICA					
PONDO	113	51	62	F. 0.259 S.E. 0.032	64
SWAZI	126	78	48	F. 0.383 S.E. 0.035	64
VENDA	80	53	27	F. 0.419 S.E. 0.046	64
XHOSA	214	129	85	F. 0.370 S.E. 0.027	64
ZULU	131	77	54	F. 0.358 S.E. 0.033	64
S.W. AFRICA					
KUAMBI OVAMBOLAND	119	62	57	F. 0.308 S.E. 0.033	64
KUANYAMA OVAMBOLAND	118	62	56	F. 0.311 S.E. 0.033	64
OKAVANGO					
BUNJA	111	62	49	F. 0.336 S.E. 0.035	64
DIRIKO	59	34	25	F. 0.349 S.E. 0.049	64
KUANGARI	47	22	25	F. 0.271 S.E. 0.050	64

TABLE XX-1 CONTINUED
TESTED FOR INV 1

		PHENOTYPES			ALLELE	
		TOTAL	1	-1	1	REF.
NEGROIDS						
AFRICA						
S.W. AFRICA						
OKAVANGO						
MBUKUSHU		115	66	49	F. 0.347 / S.E. 0.035	64
SAMBIO		98	49	49	F. 0.293 / S.E. 0.036	64
OVAHIMBA KAOKOVELD		54	27	27	F. 0.293 / S.E. 0.048	64
UPPER VOLTA						
KURUMBA		150	89	61	F. 0.362 / S.E. 0.031	57
ZAMBIA						
ILA KAFUE RIVER		41	19	22	F. 0.267 / S.E. 0.053	64
LENJE		176	101	75	F. 0.347 / S.E. 0.029	64
MLOZI ZAMBESI RIVER		189	105	84	F. 0.333 / S.E. 0.027	64
PLATEAU TONGA		120	70	50	F. 0.355 / S.E. 0.035	64
ZAMBESI VALLEY TONGA		165	88	77	F. 0.317 / S.E. 0.028	64

TABLE XX-1 CONTINUED
TESTED FOR INV 1

NEGROIDS	PHENOTYPES			ALLELE		
N. AMERICA						
U.S.A.	TOTAL	1	1-1	1		REF.
CLEVELAND, OH.	134	68	66	F. 0.298 S.E. 0.031		154
CLEVELAND, OH.	329	174	155	F. 0.314 S.E. 0.020		155

TABLE XX-2
TESTED FOR INV 2

NEGROIDS	PHENOTYPES			ALLELE		
AFRICA						
SENEGAL	TOTAL	2	2-2	2		REF.
DAKAR	399	214	185	F. 0.319 S.E. 0.018		114
OUOLOF DAKAR	173	108	65	F. 0.387 S.E. 0.030		123
PEULH DAKAR	95	45	50	F. 0.275 S.E. 0.035		123
SERERES DAKAR	129	91	38	F. 0.457 S.E. 0.037		123
TOUCOULEUR DAKAR	64	32	32	F. 0.293 S.E. 0.044		123

TABLE XX-3
TESTED FOR INV 1,2

PHENOTYPES   ALLELES

NEGROIDS

AFRICA

CENTRAL AFRICAN EMPIRE

	TOTAL	1-1	2-2		1	2	REF.
BABINGA PYGMIES	164	96	68	F.	0.356	0.644	16
				S.E.	0.030	0.030	

TABLE XX-4
TESTED FOR INV 1,3

PHENOTYPES   ALLELES

NEGROIDS

N. AMERICA

U.S.A.

		TOTAL		1	1-3	3	DF	CHI SQ. VALUE		1	3	REF.
CLAXTON, GA.		187	O.	31	85	71	1	0.419	F.	0.393	0.607	10
			E.	28.9	89.2	68.9			S.E.	0.025	0.025	
CLEVELAND, OH.		31	O.	4	15	12	1	0.042	F.	0.371	0.629	154
			E.	4.3	14.5	12.3			S.E.	0.061	0.061	
CLEVELAND, OH.		165	O.	22	74	69	1	0.094	F.	0.358	0.642	155
			E.	21.1	75.8	68.1			S.E.	0.026	0.026	

TABLE XXI-1
TESTED FOR INV 1,2

POLYNESIANS

OCEANIA

U. S. A.

	PHENOTYPES				ALLELES			
	TOTAL	1	1 -2	1 -2		1	1 2	-1 -2	REF.
HAWAIIANS HONOLULU, HI.	70	2	47	21	F.	0.025	0.427	0.548	124
					S. E.	0.018	0.049	0.050	

TABLE XXII-1
TESTED FOR INV 1

		PHENOTYPES			ALLELE	REF.
		TOTAL	1	1 – 1	1	
OTHER POPULATIONS						
AFRICA						
EGYPT						
EGYPTIANS CAIRO		245	107	138	F. 0.249 S.E. 0.021	176
SOUTH AFRICA						
CAPE COLOUREDS JOHANNESBURG		112	40	72	F. 0.198 S.E. 0.028	64
!KUBOES-COLOURED		132	49	83	F. 0.207 S.E. 0.027	175
ASIA						
MALASYIA						
NEGRITOS		48	18	30	F. 0.209 S.E. 0.044	169
PHILIPPINES						
NEGRITOS						
AGUSAN MINDANAO		93	33	60	F. 0.197 S.E. 0.031	84
BATAAN LUZON		87	39	48	F. 0.257 S.E. 0.036	84
ZAMBALES LUZON		127	38	89	F. 0.163 S.E. 0.024	84
OCEANIA						
SEYCHELLE IS.						
SEYCHELLE ISLANDERS		160	87	73	F. 0.325 S.E. 0.029	196

209

TABLE XXII-2
TESTED FOR INV 1,3

PHENOTYPES   .   ALLELES

OTHER POPULATIONS

AFRICA

ETHIOPIA

	TOTAL	1	1 3	3	CHI SQ. DF	VALUE		1	3	REF.
SIDAMO	140	O. 8	70	62	1	4.277	F.	0.307	0.693	170
		E. 13.2	59.6	67.2			S.E.	0.028	0.028	

TABLE XXIII-1
TESTED FOR A2M 1

VARIOUS RACES	PHENOTYPES			ALLELE	
	TOTAL	1	-1	1	REF.
LOCATION NOT REPORTED					
CAUCASOIDS	351	344	7	F. 0.859 S.E. 0.026	190
MONGOLOIDS					
CHINESE	50	28	22	F. 0.337 S.E. 0.053	190
JAPANESE	116	85	31	F. 0.483 S.E. 0.040	190
NEGROIDS	108	56	52	F. 0.306 S.E. 0.035	190

211

TABLE XXIII-1 CONTINUED
TESTED FOR A2M 1

VARIOUS RACES

LOCATION NOT REPORTED

ALLELE

	TOTAL		1	REF. *
CAUCASOIDS	177	F.	0.990	68
MONGOLOIDS				
CHINESE	121	F.	0.430	68
JAPANESE	163	F.	0.530	68
POLYNESIANS				
EASTER ISLAND	59	F.	0.460	68
NEGROIDS	68	F.	0.170	68

* PHENOTYPE DATA NOT PRESENTED IN REFERENCE.

212

TABLE XXIII-1 CONTINUED
TESTED FOR A2M 1

VARIOUS RACES	PHENOTYPES			ALLELE	REF.
	TOTAL	1	−1	1	
ABORIGINES					
OCEANIA					
AUSTRALIA					
BENTINCK ISLAND	46	46	0	F. 1.000 S.E. 0.074	19
MORNINGTON ISLAND	113	113	0	F. 1.000 S.E. 0.047	19
WESTERN DESERT	70	70	0	F. 1.000 S.E. 0.060	19
CAUCASOIDS					
EUROPE					
NETHERLANDS					
DUTCH	798	795	3	F. 0.939 S.E. 0.018	31
MELANESIANS					
OCEANIA					
PAP. N. GUINEA					
NEW BRITAIN					
BAINING NAN GAULIM VILLAGE	43	40	3	F. 0.736 S.E. 0.074	19
SULKA NAN MOPE VILLAGE	54	33	21	F. 0.376 S.E. 0.053	19

TABLE XXIII-1 CONTINUED
TESTED FOR A2M 1

VARIOUS RACES	PHENOTYPES TOTAL	1	−1	ALLELE 1	REF.
MELANESIANS					
OCEANIA					
PAP. N. GUINEA					
NEW BRITAIN					
TOLAI MN					
BUNAMIN VILLAGE	55	51	4	F. 0.730 S.E. 0.065	19
KOULON VILLAGE	45	21	24	F. 0.270 S.E. 0.051	19
KURAIP VILLAGE	39	31	8	F. 0.547 S.E. 0.071	19
NORDUP VILLAGE	40	26	14	F. 0.408 S.E. 0.064	19
RAKUNAI VILLAGE	17	16	1	F. 0.757 S.E. 0.118	19
RALMALMAL VILLAGE	68	51	17	F. 0.500 S.E. 0.053	19
VAIRIKI VILLAGE	56	36	20	F. 0.402 S.E. 0.054	19
VUNALAKA VILLAGE	18	15	3	F. 0.592 S.E. 0.108	19
VUNALIA VILLAGE	48	38	10	F. 0.544 S.E. 0.064	19

TABLE XXIII-1 CONTINUED
TESTED FOR AZM 1

VARIOUS RACES	PHENOTYPES			ALLELE	REF.
	TOTAL	1	—1	1	
MELANESIANS					
OCEANIA					
PAP. N. GUINEA					
NEW GUINEA					
GOGODARA NAN BALIMO VILLAGE	99	88	11	F. 0. 667 S. E. 0. 047	19
KUMAN NAN MINJ VILLAGE	101	97	4	F. 0. 801 S. E. 0. 049	19
MOTU MN POREBADA VILL.	38	19	19	F. 0. 293 S. E. 0. 057	19

TABLE XXIII-2
TESTED FOR A2M 1, 2

VARIOUS RACES

LOCATION NOT REPORTED

			PHENOTYPES		CHI SQ.		ALLELES		REF.
	TOTAL	1	1 2	2	DF	VALUE	1	2	
ABORIGINES AUSTRALIA	19	O. 17	2	0	0		F. 0.947	0.053	71
		E. 17.1	1.9	0.1			S.E. 0.036	0.036	
CAUCASOIDS	100	O. 97	3	0	0		F. 0.985	0.015	71
		E. 97.0	3.0	0.0			S.E. 0.009	0.009	
MONGOLOIDS									
AMERINDIANS	40	O. 39	1	0	0		F. 0.988	0.012	71
		E. 39.0	1.0	0.0			S.E. 0.012	0.012	
CHINESE	24	O. 0	6	18	0		F. 0.125	0.875	71
		E. 0.4	5.3	18.4			S.E. 0.048	0.048	
ESKIMOS	21	O. 16	4	1	0		F. 0.857	0.143	71
		E. 15.4	5.1	0.4			S.E. 0.054	0.054	
JAPANESE	98	O. 30	49	19	1	0.016	F. 0.556	0.444	71
		E. 30.3	48.4	19.3			S.E. 0.035	0.035	
MELANESIANS PAPUANS	48	O. 14	25	9	1	0.135	F. 0.552	0.448	71
		E. 14.6	23.7	9.6			S.E. 0.051	0.051	
NEGROIDS									
BANTUS	24	O. 1	4	19	0		F. 0.125	0.875	71
		E. 0.4	5.3	18.4			S.E. 0.048	0.048	
PYGMIES	77	O. 8	27	42	1	1.278	F. 0.279	0.721	71
		E. 6.0	31.0	40.0			S.E. 0.036	0.036	

TABLE XXIII-2 CONTINUED
TESTED FOR A2M 1,2

VARIOUS RACES		TOTAL	PHENOTYPES 1	1 2	2	CHI SQ. DF	VALUE	ALLELES 1	2	REF.
CAUCASOIDS										
EUROPE										
CZECHOSLOVAKIA										
CENTRAL BOHEMIA	O.	341	331	10	0	0		F. 0.985	0.015	146
	E.		331.1	9.9	0.1			S.E. 0.005	0.005	
ITALY										
FERRARA	O.	85	85			0		F. 0.985		100
	E.							S.E. 0.005		
SARDINIANS	O.	401	397	4	0	0		F. 0.995	0.005	100
	E.		397.0	4.0	0.0			S.E. 0.002	0.002	
MONGOLOIDS										
ASIA										
TAIWAN										
ABORIGINES	O.	300	15	119	166	1	1.172	F. 0.248	0.752	81
	E.		18.5	112.0	169.5			S.E. 0.018	0.018	
THAILAND										
THAIS	O.	200	58	95	47	1	0.444	F. 0.528	0.472	72
	E.		55.7	99.7	44.7			S.E. 0.025	0.025	
NEGROIDS										
S. AMERICA										
SURINAM										
BUSH NEGRO	O.	62	3	23	36	1	0.077	F. 0.234	0.766	71
	E.		3.4	22.2	36.4			S.E. 0.038	0.038	

217

References cited in tables

1. Abe, T. (1965). Studies on the Gm and Inv factors in Japanese individuals and families. *Keijo J. Med.* **14**, 85–9.
2. Archimandris, A., Fertakis, A., Stathopoulou, R., Kalos, A., and Angelopoulos, B. (1975). Distribution of Gm and Inv factors in two samples of the Greek population. *Acta Genet. med. Gemell.* **24**, 329–31.
3. Bajatzadeh, M. and Walter, H. (1968). Serum protein polymorphisms in Iran. *Hum. Genet.* **6**, 40–54.
4. Bajatzadeh, M. and Walter, H. (1969). Investigations on distribution of blood and serum groups in Iran. *Hum. Biol.* **41**, 401–15.
5. Bajatzadeh, M. and Walter, H. (1969). Blood and serum group typings in Koreans. *Hum. Hered.* **19**, 514–23.
6. Benabadji, M., Ruffie, J., Larrovy, G., and Vergnes, H. (1965). Étude hémotypologique des populations du Massif du Hoggar et du Plateau de l'Air. ii. Les groupes seriques. *Bull. Soc. Anthrop.* **7**, 181–4.
7. Bjarnason, O., Bjarnason, V., Edwards, J. H., Fridriksson, S., Magnusson, M., Mourant, A. E., and Tills, D. (1975). The blood groups of Icelanders. *Ann. hum. Genet.* **36**, 425–58.
8. Blanc, M., Ruffié, J., Taleb, N., and Yaffi, G. (1972). Sur la répartition des allotypes d'immunoglobulines du système Gm dans la population Kurde. *C. r. hebd. Séanc. Acad. Sci. Paris* **274**, 764–7.
9. Blanc, M., Ducos, J., and Ruffié, J. (1970). Un nouvel allotype Gm chez l'homme: le facteur Bet (marquer) racial probable. *C. r. hebd. Séanc. Acad. Sci. Paris* **271**, 145–7.
10. Blumberg, B. S., Workman, P. L., and Hirschfeld, J. (1964). Gamma globulin, group specific, and lipoprotein groups in a U.S. white and Negro population. *Nature, Lond.* **202**, 561–3.
11. Bonné, B., Gosber, M., Ashbel, S., Mourant, A. E., and Tills, D. (1971). South-Sinai Beduin. A preliminary report on their inherited blood factors. *Am. J. phys. Anthrop.* **34**, 397–408.
12. Brandtzaeg, B. and Mohr, J. (1961). On the genetics of the Gm serum system. *Acta genet.* **11**, 111–25.
13. Brazier, D. M. and Goldsmith, K. L. G. (1968). Frequency of certain Gm and Inv factors in the United Kingdom. *Nature, Lond.* **219**, 193.
14. Brown, S. M., Gajdusek, D. C., Leyshon, W. C., Steinberg, A. G., Brown, K. S., and Curtain, C. C. (1974). Genetic studies in Paraguay: blood group, red cell, and serum genetic patterns of the Guayaki and Ayore Indians, Mennonite Settlers, and seven other Indian Tribes of the Paraguayan Chaco. *Am. J. phys. Anthrop.* **41**, 317–44.
15. Carles-Trochain, E. (1968). Étude hémotypologique des pêcheurs du lac Titicaca. *Monographies du centre d'hémotypologie* Hermann, C. H. U. de Toulouse, Paris.
16. Cavalli-Sforza, L. L., Zonta, L. A., Nuzzo, F., Bernini, L., De Jong, W. W. W., Khan, P. M., Ray, A. K., Went, L. N., Siniscalco, M., Nijenhuis, L. E., van Loghem, E., and Modiano, G. (1969). Studies on African Pygmies. I. A pilot investigation of Babinga Pygmies in the Central African Republic (with an analysis of genetic distances). *Am. J. hum. Genet.* **21**, 252–74.
17. Chopra, V. P. (1970). Studies on serum groups in the Kumaon region, India. *Hum. Genet.* **10**, 35–43.
18. Curtain, C. C., van Loghem, E., Baumgarten, A., Golab, T., Gorman, J., Rutgers, C. F., and Kidson, C. (1971). The ethnological significance of the gamma-globulin (Gm) factors in Melanesia. *Am. J. phys. Anthrop.* **34**, 257–71.
19. Curtain, C. C., van Loghem, E., Fudenberg, H. H., Tindale, N. B., Simmons, R. T., Doherty, R. L., and Vos, G. (1972). Distribution of the immunoglobulin markers at the IgG1, IgG2, IgG3, IgA2 and K-chain loci in Australian Aborigines: Comparison with New Guinea populations. *Am. J. hum. Genet.* **24**, 145–55.
20. Daveau, M., Rivat, L., Langaney, A., Feingold, N., and Ropartz, C. (1975). Gm and Inv allotypes in a Gypsy sample. *Hum. Hered.* **25**, 135–43.
21. Daveau, M., Rivat, L., Langaney, A., Afifi, N., Bois, E., and Ropartz, C. (1975). Gm and Inv allotypes in French Guiana Indians. *Hum. Hered.* **25**, 88–92.
22. Deicher, von H., Wendt, G. G., Theile, U., and Kirchberg, G. (1963). Familienuntersuchungen über die Gammaglobulin gruppen Gm(a), Gm(b), Gm(x) und Gm(r). *Acta genet.* **13**, 124–31.
23. Ducos, J., Fernet, P., and Vergnes, H. (1965). Étude hémotypologique des populations du Tidikelt, les groupes sériques. *Bull. Mém. Soc. Anthrop. Paris* **7**, 185–7.
24. Durante, F., and Ronchi, G. U. (1967). Il systema Gm nella popolazione del Lazio. *Acta Genet. med. Gemell.* **16**, 190–7.
25. El Hassan, A. M., Godber, M. G., Kopeć, A. C., Mourant, A. E., Tills, D., and Lehmann, H. (1968). The hereditary blood factors of the Beja of the Sudan. *Man* **3**, 272–83.
26. Erickson, R. P., Nerlove, S., Creger, W. P., and Romney, A. K. (1970). Comparison of genetic and anthropological interpretations of population isolates in Aguacatenango, Chiapas, Mexico. *Am. J. phys. Anthrop.* **32**, 105–20.
27. Eyquem, A. and Podliachouk, L. (1963). Répartition des facteurs Gm dans certaines populations de race Noire. *Méd. trop.* **23**, 587–94.
28. Fernet, P., Larrouy, C., and Ruffié, J. (1964). Étude hémotypologique des populations Indiennes de Guyane Française II. Les groupes sériques du système Gm. *Bull. Mém. Soc. Anthropol. Paris* **7**, 119–23.
29. Flory, L. L. (1964). Serum factors of Australian Aborigines from North Queensland. *Nature, Lond.* **201**, 508–9.
30. Fraser, G. R., Grünwald, P., Kitchin, F. D., and Steinberg, A. G. (1969). Serum polymorphisms in Yugoslavia. *Hum. Hered,* **19**, 57–64.
31. Fraser, G. R., Volkers, W. S., Bernin, L. F., van Loghem, E., Meera Kahn, P., and Nijenhuis, L. E. (1974). Gene frequencies in a Dutch population. *Hum. Hered.* **24**, 435–48.
32. Fraser, G. R., Steinberg, A. G., Defaranas, B., Mayo, O., Stamatoyannopoulos, G., and Motulsky, A. G. (1969). Gene frequencies at loci determining blood group and serum protein polymorphisms in two villages of Northwestern Greece. *Am. J. hum. Genet.* **21**, 46–60.
33. Friedlaender, J. S., and Steinberg, A. G. (1970). Anthropological significance of gamma globulin (Gm and Inv) antigens in Bougainville Island, Melanesia. *Nature, Lond.* **228**, 59–61.
34. Gallango, M. L. and Arends, T. (1965). Inv(2) serum factor in Venezuelan Indians. *Transfusion* **5**, 457–60.
35. Gedde-Dahl, T. and Berg, K. (1965). Linkage in man: the Inv and the Lp serum type systems. *Nature, Lond.* **208**, 1126.
36. Gedde-Dahl, T., Jr., Natvig, J. B., and Gundersen, S. K. (1971). Inheritance of Gm(g) and a gene complex Gm^{a}Gm$^{g\ weak}$. *Clin. Genet.* **2**, 356–66.
37. Geerdink, R. A., Nijenhuis, L. E., van Loghem, E., Sjoe, E. L. F. (1974). Blood groups and immunoglobulin groups in Trio and Wajana Indians from Surinam. *Am. J. hum. Genet.* **26**, 45–53.
38. Gessain, R., Ruffié, J., Kane, Y., Kane, O., Cabannes, R., and Gomila, J. (1965). Note sur la sero-anthropologie de trois populations de Guinée et du Senegal: Coniagui, Bassari, et Bedik. *Bull. Mém. Soc. Anthrop. Paris* XI serie, 5–18.
39. Gessain, R., Moullec, J., and Gomila, J. (1965). Groupes d'haptoglobine et du transferrins et groupes Gm des Coniagui et

218

des Bassari. *Bull. Soc. Anthrop., Paris* **8**, 19–22.

40. GILES, E., OGAN, E., and STEINBERG, A. G. (1965). Gamma-globulin factors (Gm and Inv) in New Guinea: anthropological significance. *Science, Wash.* **150**, 1158–60.

41. GODBER, M. J., KOPEĆ, A. C., MOURANT, A. E., TILLS, D., and LEHMANN, E. E. (1973). The hereditary blood factors of the Yemenite and Kurdish Jews. *Phil. Trans. R. Soc. Lond.* **266**, 169–84.

42. GODBER, M., KOPEĆ, A. C., MOURANT, A. E., TEESDALE, P., TILLS, D., WEINER, J. S., EL-NEIL, H., WOOD, C. H., and BARLEY, S. (1976). The blood groups, serum proteins, red cell enzymes and haemoglobulins of Sandawe and Nyatura of Tanzania. *Ann. hum. Biol.* **3**, 463–73.

43. GÖHLER, W., DÜRWALD, W., and HUNGER, H. (1963). Gm-frequenzen und Verwertbarkeit des Gm-systems in Paternitätsgutachten. *Dt. Z. ges. gericht. Med.* **53**, 122–30.

44. GÖHLER, W. (1970). Untersuchungen zur Populations-und Formalgenetik des Gm-systems im Raum Leipzig. *Arch. Kriminol.* **146**, 40–57.

45. GÖHLER, W. (1967). Untersuchungen zur Faktoren-und Phänotypenhäufigkeit im Gm-system bei einigen aussereuropäischen Populationen. *Z. ärztl. Fortbild.* **61**, 773–6.

46. HALLBERG, T. (1968). Gm(1), (Gm(2), Gm(4) and Gm(5) in a Korean population. *Acta genet.* **18**, 468–74.

47. HARBOE, M. and LUNDEVALL, J. (1961). The application of the Gm system in paternity cases. *Vox Sang.* **6**, 257–73.

48. HARRISON, G. A., KÜCHEMANN, C. F., MOORE, M. A. S., BOYCE, A. J., BAJU, T., MOURANT, A. E., GODBER, M. J., GLASGOW, B. G., KOPEĆ, A. C., TILLS, D., and CLEGG, E. J. (1969). The effects of altitudinal variation in Ethiopian populations. *Phil. Trans. R. Soc.* **256**, 147–82.

49. HERZOG, P. and DRDOVÁ, A. (1961). Inv factor in CSSR. *Vox Sang.* **6**, 636–7.

50. HERZOG, P. and KOUT, M. (1963). Praktische Anwendung der Serumgruppen in Paternitätsprozessen. *Dt. Z. ges. Gerichts. Med.* **53**, 186–94.

51. HERZOG, P. and HUNGER, H. (1964). Frequenz-und Familienuntersuchungen über die Verteilung des Faktors Inv(a) in der tschechischen und mitteldeutschen Bevölkerung. *Z. mensch. Vererb.- u. Konstitlehre* **37**, 626–31.

52. HERZOG, P. and CORONA, P. O. G. (1967). Hp-, Gm-, Inv- und Tf-typen in Santiago de Cuba (Cuba). (1967). *Folia haemat.* **87**, 260–6.

53. HERZOG, P., BOHATOVÁ, J. and DRDOVÁ, A. (1970). Genetic polymorphisms in Kenya. *Am. J. hum. Genet.* **22**, 287–91.

54. HERZOG, P., DRDOVÁ, A., and BOHATOVÁ, J. (1976). Serum polymorphisms in North Vietnam. *Hum. Hered.* **26** 203–6.

55. HIERNAUX, J. (1976). Blood polymorphism frequencies in the Sara Majingay of Chad. *Ann. hum. Biol.* **3**, 127–40.

56. HILL, Z., MAKEŠOVÁ, D., and KREWJČOVÁ, O. (1968). The factors Gm(1), Gm(2), Gm(4), Gm(5), and Inv(1) in the sera of patients with allergic diseases. *Acta allerg.* **23**, 124–9.

57. HUIZINGA, J. (1969). Human biological observations on some African populations of the Thorn Savanna Belt II. *Proc. k. Ned. Akad. Wet.* C **71**, 373–90.

58. HUMMEL, K., PULVERER, G., SCHAAL, K. P., and WEIDTMAN, V. (1970). Häufigkeit der Sichttypen in den Erbsystemen Haptoglobin, Gc, saure Erythrocytenphosphatase, Phosphoglucomutase und Adenylatkinase sowie den Erbeigenschaften Gm(1), Gm(2), und Inv(1) bei Deutschen (aus dem Raum Freiburg i. Br. und Köln) und bei Türken. *Hum. Genet.* **8**, 330–3.

59. HUNGER, H., GÖHLER, W., and DÜRWALD, W. (1963). Familienuntersuchungen im Gm-system. *Vox Sang.* **8**, 86–9.

60. HUNGER, H. and HERZOG, P. (1965). Examinations of the Inv(a) factor in families. *Vox Sang.* **10**, 635–7.

61. IZATT, M. ABO and Gm phenotypes found North of Scotland. Personal communication.

62. JENKINS, T. and STEINBERG, A. G. (1966). Some serum protein polymorphisms in Kalahari Bushman and Bantu: gamma globulins, haptoglobins and transferrins. *Am. J. hum. Genet.* **18**, 399–407.

63. JENKINS, T. and BRAIN, C. K. (1967). The peoples of the lower Kuiseb valley, South West Africa. *Scient. Pap. Namib Desert Res. Stn,* **35**.

64. JENKINS, T., ZOUTENDYK, A., and STEINBERG, A. G. (1970). Gammaglobulin groups (Gm and Inv) of various Southern African populations. *Am. J. phys. Anthrop.* **32**, 197–218.

65. KHERUMIAN, R., MOULLEC, J., and VAN CONG, N. (1967). Groupes sanguins erythrocytaires A₁A₂BO, MN, Rh(CcDE) et sériques Hp, Tf, Gm, dans quatre régions militaires Françaises. *Bull. Mém. Soc. Anthrop. Paris* **1**, 377–84.

66. KIRK, R. L., LAI, L. Y. C., VOS, G. H., WICKREMASINGHE, R., and PERERA, D. J. B. (1962). The blood and serum groups of selected populations in South India and Ceylon. *Am. J. phys. Anthrop.* **20**, 485–97.

67. KLEMPERER, M. R., HOLBROOK, E. R., and FUDENBERG, H. H. (1966). Gm(20), a new hereditary gamma globulin factor. *Am. J. hum. Genet.* **18**, 433–7.

68. KUNKEL, H. G., SMITH, W. K., JOSLIN, F. G., NATVIG, J. B., and LITWIN, S. D. (1969). Genetic marker of the γA2 subgroup of γA immunoglobulins. *Nature, Lond.* **223**, 1247–8.

69. VAN LOGHEM, E. and MÅRTENSSON, L. (1967). Genetic (Gm) determinants of the γ2c (Vi) subclass of human IgG immunoglobulins. *Vox Sang.* **13**, 369–92.

70. VAN LOGHEM, E., NATVIG, J. B., and MATSUMOTO, H. (1970). Genetic markers of immunoglobulins in Japanese families. *Ann. hum. Genet.* **33**, 351–9.

71. VAN LOGHEM, E., WANG, A. C., and SHUSTER, J. (1973). A new genetic marker of human immunoglobulins determined by an allele at the α2 locus. *Vox Sang.* **24**, 481–8.

72. VAN LOGHEM, E., CHANDANAYINGYONG, D., and DOUGLAS, R. (1975). Immunoglobulin genetic markers in the Thai population. *J. Immunogenet.* **2**, 141–5.

73. LOPEZ, V. and BÜTLER, R. (1965). The Inv groups in Switzerland. *Vox Sang.* **10**, 314–19.

74. MÅRTENSSON, L. (1964). On the relationships between the γ-globulin genes of the Gm system. *J. exp. Med.* **120**, 1169–88.

75. MÅRTENSSON, L., VAN LOGHEM, E., MATSUMOTO, H., and NIELSEN, J. (1966). Gm(s) and Gm(t): genetic determinants of human γ-globulin. *Vox Sang.* **11**, 393–418.

76. MARZIANO, E. (1968). Distribuzione dei fattori serici gruppo-specifici Gm(a), Gm(b), Gm(x) nella popalazione della Sicilia Orientale. *Medna leg.* **16**, 23–32.

77. MATSUMOTO, H. and TAKATSUKI, K. (1968). Gm factors in Japan: population and family studies. *Jap. J. hum. Genet.* **13**, 10–19.

78. MATSUMOTO, H. and TAKATSUKI, K. (1968). Studies on the Gm factors of Japanese population and families. *Jap. J. leg. Med.* **22**, 635–42.

79. MATSUMOTO, H., MIYAZAKI, T., FONG, J. M., and MABUCHI, Y. (1972). Gm and Inv allotypes of the Takasago tribes in Taiwan. *Jap. J. hum. Genet.* **17**, 27–37.

80. MATSUMOTO, H. and MIYAZAKI, T. (1972). Gm and Inv allotypes of the Ainu in Hidaka area, Hokkaido. *Jap. J. hum. Genet.* **17**, 20–6.

81. MATSUMOTO, H., MAIYAZAKI, T., and FONG, J. M. (1973). Further data on the Gm and Am allotypes of the Takasago in Taiwan. *Jap. J. leg. Med.* **27**, 273–7.

82. MATSUMOTO, H., MIYAZAKI, T., LIN, J. Y., and HOTTA, S. (1975). The serum protein groups of Indonesians from Java. *Jap. J. hum. Genet.* **20**, 201–5.

83. MATSUMOTO, H., MIYAZAKI, T., and LIN, J. (1975). Gm and Km allotypes of the Taiwanese. *Jap. J. hum. Genet.* **20**, 169–73.

84. MATSUMOTO, H., MIYAZAKI, T., OMOTO, K., MISAWA, S., HARADA, S., SUMPAICO, J. S., MEDADO, P. M., and OYONUKI, H. Population genetic studies of the Philippine Negritos. II. Gm and Inv allotypes of three population groups. Personal communication.

85. MATZNETTER, T. and SPIELMANN, W. (1969). Blutgruppen mocambiquanischer Bantustämme. *Z. Morph. Anthrop.* **61**, 57–71,

86. MAYR, W. R. and MICKERTS, D. (1970). Der menschliche gammaglobulin polymorphismus. *Acta biol. med. germ.* **25**, 473–482.

87. MCALPINE, P. J., CHEN, S. H. COX, D. W., DOSSETOR, J. B., GIBLETT, E., STEINBERG, A. G., and SIMPSON, N. E. (1974). Genetic markers in blood in a Canadian Eskimo population with a comparison of allele frequencies in circumpolar populations. *Hum. Hered.* **24**, 114–42.

88. MOULLEC, J., RUFFIÉ, J., MATTE, C., AUDRAN, R., and NOEL, M. (1961). Observations sur la Répartition des groupes sériques (haptoglobines, transferrine, groupes Gm) dans quelques populations. *Proc. 2nd Int. Cong. hum. Genet.* **II**, 762–5.

89. MOURANT, A. E., GODBER, M. J., KOPEĆ, A. C., LEHMANN, H., STEELE, P. R., and TILLS, D. (1968). The hereditary blood factors of some populations in Bhutan. *The Anthropologist* special volume: 29–43.

90. NAKAJIMA, H. and OHKURA, K. (1971). The distribution of several serological and biochemical traits in East Asia II. The distribution of gamma-globulin [Gm(1),

Gm(2), Gm(5), and Inv (1)] and Gc groups in Taiwan and Ryukyu. *Hum. Hered.* **21**, 362–70.

91. NEEL, J. V., SALZANO, F. M., JUNQUEIRA, P. C., KEITER, F., and MAYBURY-LEWIS, D. (1964). Studies on the Xavante Indians of the Brazilian Mato Grossa. *Am, J. hum. Genet.* **16**, 52–140.

92. NICHOLLS, E. M., LEWIS, H. B. M., COOPER, D. W., and BENNETT, J. H. (1965). Blood group and serum protein differences in some Central Australian Aborigines. *Am. J. hum. Genet.* **17**, 293–307.

93. NIELSEN, J. C. (1961). Studies on the inheritance of the Gm groups. *Proc. 2nd Int. Congr. human. Genet.* **II**, 766–70.

94. NIELSEN, J. C., MÅRTENSSON, L., GÜRTLER, H., GILBERT, Å., and TINGSGÅRD, P. (1971). Gm types of Greenland Eskimos. *Hum. Hered.* **21**, 405–19.

95. PÁLSSON, J. and WALTER, H. (1967). Untersuchungen zur Populationsgenetik von Island, insbesondere der Region Dalasýsla. *Hum. genet.* **4**, 352–61.

96. PÁLSSON, J. O. P., WALTER, H., and BAJAT-ZADEH, M. (1970). Serogenetical studies in Ireland. *Hum. Hered.* **20**, 231–9.

97. PEREIRA, T. M. and MANSO, C. (1975). Immunoglobulin allotypes in Portugal. *Hum. Genet.* **27**, 137–40.

98. PERSSON, I., RIVAT, L., ROUSSEAU, P. Y., and ROPARTZ, C. (1972). Ten Gm factors and the Inv system in Eskimos in Greenland. *Hum. Hered.* **22**, 519–28.

99. PHANSOMBOON, S. and SINGHPRASERT, P., (1970). The Gm and Inv factors of the Thai people. *Vox Sang.* **18**, 274–6.

100. PIAZZA, A., VAN LOGHEM, E., DE LANGE, G., CURTONI, E. S., ULIZZI, L., and TERRENATO, L. (1976). Immunoglobulin allotypes in Sardinia. *Am. J. hum. Genet.* **28**, 77–86.

101. PODLIACHOUK, L., EYQUEM, A., CHOARIPOUR, R., and EFTEKHARI, M. (1962). Les facteurs sériques Gm(a), Gm(b), Gm(x) et Gm-like chez les Iraniens. *Vox Sang.* **7**, 496–9.

102. PODLIACHOUK, L. and EYQUEM, A. (1963). Les facteurs sériques Gm(a), Gm(b), Gm(x) et Gm-like dans la race blanche. *C.r. séanc. Soc. biol.* **157**, 732–6.

103. PROKOP, O. and ANASTASOW, B. (1966). Familiendaten zur Vererbung von Gm(f). *Dte. Gesundh Wes.* **21** 1027–8.

104. PROKOP, O. and ANASTASOW, B. (1966). Familiendaten zur Vererbung von Inv(1). *Dte. GesundhWes.* **21**, 1028.

105. QUILICI, J. C., RUFFIÉ, J., and MARTY, Y. (1970). Hémotypologie d'un groupe paléo-amérindien des Andes: les Chipaya. *Nouv. Revue fr. Hémat.* **10**, 727–38.

106. REED, T. E. (1969). Critical tests of hypotheses for race mixture using Gm data on American Caucasians and Negroes. *Am. J. hum. Genet.* **21**, 71–83.

107. REX-KISS, B. and HORVATH, E. (1971). Ergebnisse der Blut-und Serumgruppen-Bestimmungen in Ungarn (Phänotypen-, Genotypen-und Genfrequenzen). *Z. Immun.Forsch. exp. Ther.* **141**, 449–59.

108. RITTER, H., ROPARTZ, C., ROUSSEAU, P. Y. RIVAT, L., and SATI, A. (1964). Studies on the formal genetics of the gammaglobulin polymorphism Gm [characters Gm(a), Gm(b), Gm(x)]. *Vox Sang.* **9**, 340–8.

109. RITTER, H., ROPARTZ, C., ROUSSEAU, P. Y., RIVAT, L., and BÄHR, M. L. (1964). Zur Formalgenetik und Populationsgenetik des Gammaglobulin-Polymorphisms Inv [Merkmale Inv(1) und Inv(2)]. *Acta genet.* **14**, 15–24.

110. RITTER, H. and DRESCHER, K. H. (1964). Bestimmungstechnik der Gammaglobulin-Polymorphismen Gm und Inv. *Das Ärztliche Laboratorium* **10**, 88–97.

111. RITTER, H. and WENDT, G. G. (1964). Untersuchung von 223 Familien zur formalen Genetik des INV-Polymorphismus. *Hum. Genet.* **1**, 123–5.

112. RITTER, H. and SCHMIDTMANN, E. (1964). Das Anti-Inv-1-Rie. *Hum. Genet.* **1**, 144–8.

113. RITTER, H., ROPARTZ, C., ROUSSEAU, P. Y., RIVAT, L., and WALTER, H. (1966). Formale Genetik und Populations Genetik des Inv-Polymorphismus. *Z. Blutforschung* **13**, 373–7.

114. ROPARTZ, C., RIVAT, L., and LENOIR, J. (1960). Fréquence des facteurs Gma, Gmb, Gmx, Gm-like et Inv chez quatre cents Noires Africans. *Rev. Franç. D'Études Clin. et Biol.* **5**, 814–16.

115. ROPARTZ, C., RIVAT, L., ROUSSEAU, P. Y., and LENOIR, J. (1961). Les facteurs Gma, Gmb, Gmx, "Gm-like" et Inv chez les Japonais. *Rev. fr. Étud. clin. biol.* **6**, 813–16.

116. ROPARTZ, C., LENOIR, J., and RIVAT, L. (1961). A new inheritable property of human sera: the inV factor. *Nature, Lond.* **189**, 586.

117, ROPARTZ, C., ROUSSEAU, P. Y., RIVAT, L., and LENOIR, J. (1961). Étude génetique du facteur sérique Inv fréquence dans certaines populations. *Rev. fr. Étud. clin. biol.* **6**, 374–7.

118. ROPARTZ, C., RUFFIÉ, J., DUCOS, J., and RIVAT, L. (1961). Sur la répartition des groupes sériques dans les populations de la Saoura (Sahara occidental). *C. r. Soc. Biol.* **155**, 1589–90.

119. ROPARTZ, C., RIVAT, L., ROUSSEAU, P. Y., CHOARIPOUR, R., and EFTEKHARI, M. (1962). Répartition des groupes de gammag-lobulines: Gm et Inv chez les Iraniens. *Acta genet.* **12**, 45–50.

120. ROPARTZ, C., ROUSSEAU, P. Y., and RIVAT, L. (1962). Le système de γ-globuline, Gm, dans une population de la Seine-Maritime, fréquence des phénotypes. Études familiale. *Rev. fr. Étud. clin. biol.* **7**, 847–55.

121. ROPARTZ, C., ROUSSEAU, P. Y., RIVAT, L., and KIRK, R. L. (1962). Fréquence du facteur Inv(2) chez les Aborigines de L'ouest Australien. *Nouv. Revue fr. Hémat.* **2**, 86–90.

122. ROPARTZ, C., RIVAT, L., ROUSSEAU, P. V., BAITSCH, H., and VAN LOGHEM, J. (1963). Les Systèmes Gm et Inv en Europe. *Acta genet.* **13**, 109–23.

123. ROPARTZ, C., ROUSSEAU, P. Y., and RIVAT, L. (1963). Intérêt des groupes de γ-globuline Gm et Inv dans l'appréciation du métissage des Populations: Étude de ces groupes sériques dans l'ouest Africain et l'extrême-orient. *Rev. fr. Étud. clin. biol.* **8**, 465–72.

124. ROPARTZ, C., ROUSSEAU, P. Y., RIVAT, L., BAITSCH, H., RITTER, H., PINKERTON, F. J.,

and MERMOD, L. E., (1964). Les groupes de gamma-globulines Gm et Inv parmi la population d'Honolulu (Hawaii). *Acta genet.* **14**, 25–35.

125. ROPARTZ, C., WALTER, H., ARNDT-HANSER, A., RIVAT, L., ROUSSEAU, P. Y., and BERNHARD, W. (1964). On the frequency of the Gm- and Inv-Serum groups in South-Western Germany. *Acta genet.* **14**, 298–308.

126. ROPARTZ, C., ROUSSEAU, P. Y., and RIVAT, L. (1965). Hypothéses sur la génétique formelle du système Gm chez les Caucasiens. *Hum. Genet.* **1**, 483–96.

127. ROPARTZ, C., RIVAT, L., ROUSSEAU, P. Y., and FINE, J. M. (1965). Myélomes, maladies de Waldenström et groupes de gamma-globulines Gm et Inv. *Rev. fr. Étud. clin. biol.* **10**, 507–13.

128. ROPARTZ, C., Gold, E. R., RIVAT, L., and ROUSSEAU, P. Y. (1966). Fréquence du facteur Gm(4) parmi quelques populations blanches, noires et jaunes. *Transfusion* (Paris) **9**, 293–301.

129. ROPARTZ, C., ROUSSEAU, P. Y., RIVAT, L., and RIVAT, C. (1967). Un nouveau facteur du système Gm: le Gm(18). *Rev. fr. étud. clin. biol.* **12**, 443–51.

130. ROPARTZ, C., RIVAT, L., ROUSSEAU, P. Y., WALTER, H., and NEMESKÉRI, J. (1968). Observations on the distribution of the Gm- and Inv- groups in Hungary. *Hum. Genet.* **5**, 165–9.

131. ROPARTZ, C., RIVAT, L., ROUSSEAU, P. Y., LAURIDSEN, B., and PERSSON, I. (1970). A survey of 9 Gm-factors, the Inv and the Isf systems in Danes. *Hum. Hered.* **20**, 456–61.

132. ROPARTZ, C., RIVAT, L., ROUSSEAU, P. Y., and LEGUEULT, L. C. (1972). Frequency of Gm, Inv and Isf phenotypes in the population of 4 Yugoslavian villages. *Hum. Hered.* **22**, 508–18.

133. RUFFIÉ, J., CABANNES, R., and LARROUY, G. (1962). Étude hémotypologique des populations Berbères de M'Sirda-Fouaga (Nord-Quest Oranais). *Bull. Mém. Soc. Antrhop. Paris* **3**, 294–314.

134. RUFFIÉ, J., FERNET, P., and DURRIEU-VARSI, M. (1964). Possibilités de quatre gènes principaux: Gm(a), Gm(b), Gm(ax), Gm(ab) dans les populations Caucasoïdes. *C.r. hebd. Séanc. Acad. Sc. Paris* **259**; 2147–8.

135. RUFFIÉ, J. and TALEB, N. (1965). Étude hémotypologique des ethnies Libanaises. *Monogrs. Cent. Hématypologie.*

136. RUFFIÉ, J., LARROUY, G., and VERGNES, H. (1966). Hématologie comparée des populations Amérindiennes de Bolivie et phénomènes adaptatifs. *Nouv. Revue fr. Hémat.* **6**, 544–52.

137. SALZANO, F. M. and STEINBERG, A. G. (1965). The Gm and Inv groups of Indians from Santa Caterina, Brazil. *Am. J. hum. Genet.* **17**, 273–9.

138. SALZANO, F. M., STEINBERG, A. G., and TEPFENHART, M. A. (1973). Gm and Inv allotypes of Brazilian Cayapo Indians. *Am. J. hum. Genet.* **25**, 167–77.

139. SCHANFIELD, M. S. (1971). Population studies on the Gm and Inv antigens in Asia and Oceania. Ph.D. Thesis, library of University of Michigan, pp. 1–137. Data published in part in Ref. 140.

140. SCHANFIELD, M. S., GILES, E., and

GERSHOWITZ, H. (1975). Genetic studies in the Markham Valley, Northeastern Papua New Guinea: gamma globulin (Gm and Inv), group specific component (Gc) and ceruloplasmin (Cp) typing. *Am. J. phys. Anthrop.* **42**, 1–8.

141. SCHANFIELD, M. S. and GERSHOWITZ, H. (1971). Studies on the immunoglobulin allotypes of Asiatic populations I. Gm and Inv allotypes among Chinese from Kuantung Province. *Hum. Hered.* **21**, 168–72.

142. SCHANFIELD, M. S., GERSHOWITZ, H., OHKURA, K., and BLACKWELL, R. Q. (1972). Studies on the immunoglobulin allotypes of Asiatic populations II. Gm and Inv allotypes in Chinese. *Hum. Hered.* **22**, 138–43.

143. SCHANFIELD, M. S., GERSHOWITZ, H., HONG, K.-J., and SHIM, B.-S. (1972). Studies on the immunoglobulin allotypes of Asiatic populations III. Gm and Inv allotypes among random Koreans. *Hum. Hered.* **22**, 144–8.

144. SCHANFIELD, M. S., GERSHOWITZ, H., and OHKURA, K. (1972). Studies on the immunoglobulin allotypes of Asiatic populations IV. Gm and Inv allotypes in three Japanese prefectures and Okinawa. *Hum. Hered.* **22**, 496–502.

145. SCHANFIELD, M. S., GERGELY, J., and FUNDENBERG, H. H. (1975). Immunoglobulin allotypes in European populations I. Gm and Km (Inv) allotypic markers in Hungarians. *Hum. Hered.* **25**, 370–7.

146. SCHANFIELD, M. S., HERZOG, P., and FUDENBERG, H. H. (1975). Immunoglobulin allotypes of European populations. II. Gm, Am, and Km (Inv) allotypic markers in Czechoslovakia. *Hum. Hered.* **25**, 382–92.

147. SCHLESINGER, D. (1968). The Inv(1) factor in the Polish population. *Arch. Immunol. Ther. exp.* **16**, 742–6.

148. SCHLESINGER, D. and LUCZKIEWICZ-MULCZYKOWA, A. (1971). The Gm(1), Gm(2) and Gm(4) factors in the Polish population. *Arch. Immunol. Ther. exp.* **19**, 703–708.

149. SEEMANOVA, E., KUBICKOVA, Z., KOUT, M., and HERZOG, P. (1972). Krevni Skupiny Ve Dvou Vychadoslovenskych Izolatech. *Bratisl. lek. Listy* 57c 1 Januar.

150. SHREFFLER, D. C. and STEINBERG, A. G. (1967). Further studies on the Xavante Indians IV. Serum protein groups and the SC trait of saliva in the Simões Lopes and São Marcos Xavantes. *Am. J. hum. Genet.* **19**, 514–23.

151. SOCHA, W. and KACZERA, Z. (1968). Studies on the gamma-globulin group systems in the Polish population. *Folia biol. Kraków* **16**, 145–65.

152. STEINBERG, A. G., LAI, L. Y. C., VOS, G. H., BHAGWAN SINGH, R., and LIM, T. W. (1961). Genetic and population studies of the blood types and serum factors among Indians and Chinese from Malaya. *Am. J. hum. Genet.* **13**, 355–71.

153. STEINBERG, A. G., STAUFFER, R., BLUMBERG, B. S., and FUDENBERG, H. (1961). Gm phenotypes and genotypes in U.S. whites and Negroes; in American Indians and Eskimos; in Africans; and in Micronesians. *Am. J. hum. Genet.* **13**, 205–13.

154. STEINBERG, A. G. (1962). Progress in the study of genetically determined human gamma globulin types (the Gm and Inv groups). *Prog. med. Genet.* **2**, 1–33.

155. STEINBERG, A. G., WILSON, J. A., and LANSET, S. (1962). A new human gamma globulin factor determined by an allele at the Inv locus. *Vox Sang.* **7**, 151–6.

156. STEINBERG, A. G. and WILSON, J. A. (1963). Studies on heriditary gamma globulin factors: evidence that Gm(b) in whites and Negroes is not the same and that Gm-like is determined by an allele at the Gm locus. *Am. J. hum. Genet.* **15**, 96–105.

157. STEINBERG, A. G. and MATSUMOTO, H. (1964). Studies on the Gm, Inv, Hp and Tf serum factors of Japanese populations and families. *Hum. Biol.* **36**, 77–85.

158. STEINBERG, A. G. and GOLDBLUM, R. (1965). A genetic study of the antigens associated with the Gm(b) factor of human gamma globulin. *Am. J. hum. Genet.* **17**, 133–47.

159. STEINBERG and KIRK — unpublished data on Australian Aborigines. Quoted by Kirk 'The distribution of genetic markers in Australian Aborigines.' 1965.

160. STEINBERG and GREENWALT. Unpublished data.

161. STEINBERG and RUCKNAGEL. Unpublished data.

162. STEINBERG, A. G. (1966). Letters to the Editor: Correction of previously published Gm(c) phenotypes of Africans and Micronesians. *Am. J. hum. Genet.* **18**, 109.

163. STEINBERG, A. G. (1966). Gm and Inv studies of a Hokkaido population: evidence for a Gm^2 allele in the Ainu. *Am. J. hum. Genet.* **18**, 459–66.

164. STEINBERG, A. G., CORDOVA, M. S., and LISKER, R. (1967). Studies on several hematologic traits of Mexicans XV. The Gm allotypes of some Indian tribes. *Am. J. hum. Genet.* **19**, 747–56.

165. STEINBERG, A. G. and KAGEYAMA, S. (1970). Further data on the Gm and Inv allotypes of the Ainu: confirmation of the presence of a $Gm^{2,17,21}$ phenogroup. *Am. J. hum. Genet.* **22**, 319–25.

166. STEINBERG, A. G. and KIRK, R. L. (1970). Gm and Inv types of Aborigines in the Northern Territory of Australia. *Archaeol. & Phys. Anthrop. Oceania* **5**, 163–72.

167. STEINBERG, A. G., DAMON, A, and BLOOM, J. (1972). Gammaglobulin allotypes of Melanesians from Malaita and Bougainville, Solomon Islands. *Am. J. phys. Anthrop.* **36**, 77–84.

168. STEINBERG, A. G., GAJDUSEK, D. C., and ALPERS, M. (1972). Genetic studies in relation to Kuru. V. Distribution of human gamma globulin allotypes in New Guinea populations. *Am. J. hum. Genet.* **24**, S95–S110.

169. STEINBERG, A. G. and LIE-INJO LUAN ENG. (1972). Immunoglobulin G allotypes in Malayan Aborigines. *Hum. Hered.* **22**, 254–8.

170. STEINBERG, A. G. (1973). Gm and Inv allotypes of some Sidamo Ethiopians. *Am. J. Phys. Anthrop.* **39**, 403–8.

171. STEINBERG, A. G. (1973). The Gm and Inv allotypes of some Ashkenazic Jews living in Northern U.S.A. *Am. J. phys. Anthrop.* **39**, 409–12.

172. STEINBERG, A. G. and MORTON, N. E. (1973). Immunoglobulins in the Eastern Carolinas. *Am. J. phys. Anthrop.* **38**, 699–702.

173. STEINBERG, A. G., UNDEVIA, J. V., and TEPFENHART, M. A. (1973). Gm and Inv studies of Parsi and Irani in India: report of a new polymorphic haplotype, $Gm^{1,3,21}$. *Am. J. hum. Genet.* **25**, 302–9.

174. STEINBERG, A. G., TIILIKAINEN, A., ESKOLA, M. R., and ERIKSSON, A. W. (1974). Gammaglobulin allotypes in Finnish Lapps, Finns, Åland Islanders, Maris (Cheremis), and Greenland Eskimos. *Am. J. hum. Genet,* **26**, 223–43.

175. STEINBERG, A. G., JENKINS, T., NURSE, G. T., HARPENDING, H. C. (1975). Gammaglobulin groups of the Khoisan peoples of Southern Africa: evidence for polymorphism for a $Gm^{1,5,13,14,21}$ haplotype among the San. *Am. J. hum. Genet.* **27**, 528–42.

176. STEINBERG, A. G., HOUSER, H., and KHOLI. Unpublished data.

177. STEINBERG, A. G. and McGREGOR, I. A. Unpublished data.

178. STEINBERG, A. G. and MORELL, A. Unpublished data.

179. SZATHMARY, E. J. E., COX, D. W., GERSHOWITZ, H., RUCKNAGEL, D. L., and SCHANFIELD, M. S. (1974). The Northern and Southeastern Ojibwa: serum proteins and red cell enzyme systems. *Am. J. phys. Anthrop.* **40**, 49–66.

180. TALEB, N. and RUFFIÉ, J. (1968). Hémotypologie des populations Jordaniennes. *Bull. Mém. Soc. Anthrop. Paris* **3**, 269–82.

181. TIILIKAINEN, A,. ERIKSSON, A. W., and FORSIUS, H. (1964). Hereditary serum factors Gm(a), Gm(x), and Gm(b) in Finland. *Ann. Med. exp. Fenn.* **42**, 48–9.

182. TOHRU, A. (1965). Studies on the Gm and Inv factors in Japanese individuals and families. *Keijo J. Med.* **14**, 85–9.

183. UENO, N. and YOKOYAMA, M. (1964). Population study of gamma globulin types in Japanese. *Z. Immun. Allerg. Forsch.* **127**, 58–63.

184. UENO, S. (1975). Further studies on the inheritance of Gm(m) in Japanese families. *Jap. J. hum. Genet.* **19**, 317–23.

185. VAN HUNG, N. (1968). Untersuchungen zur Frequenz der Faktoren Gm(a), Gm(x), Gm(f) und Inv(1) in Vietnam. *Folia Haemat.* **89**, 80–4.

186. VIERUCCI, A. (1965). Gm groups and anti-Gm antibodies in children with Cooley's anemia. *Vox Sang.* **10**, 82–93.

187. VOGEL, F., KRÜGER, J., CHAKRAVARTTI, M. R., FLATZ, G., and RITTER, H. (1971). Inv phenotypes and quantitative gamma globulin determinations in leprosy patients and control populations from India and Thailand. *Hum. Genet.* **12**, 35–41.

188. VOS, G. H., KIRK, R. L., and STEINBERG, A. G. (1963). The distribution of the gamma globulin types Gm(a), Gm(b), Gm(x) and Gm-like in South and Southeast Asia and Australia. *Am. J. hum. Genet.* **15**, 44–52.

189. VOS, G. H., FUDENBERG, H. H., ENG, L. I. L., and STENHOUSE, N. S. (1967). A study of various antibodies and genetically determined serum groups among aborters produc-

ing anti-Tja-like hemolysis and non-aborters in Western Australia. *Acta haemat*. **38**, 231–9.

190. VYAS, G. N. and FUDENBERG, H. H. (1969). Am(1) the first genetic marker of human immunoglobulin A. *Proc. natn. Acad. Sci. U.S.A.* **64**, 1211–16.

191. WALTER, H., BERNHARD, W., HASSAN, S. T., and BAJATZADEH, M. (1966). Untersuchungen über die Verteilung der Hp-, Gc- und Gm-Gruppen in Pakistan. *Hum. Genet.* **2**, 262–70.

192. WALTER, H. and NEMESKÉRI, J. (1967). Demographical and sero-genetical studies on the population of Bodrogköz (NE Hungary). *Hum. Biol.* **39**, 224–40.

193. WALTER, H. and YANNISSIS, C. (1967). Zur Häufigkeit der Serumproteinpolymorphismen Hp, Gc, Gm, Inv und Lp in Griechenland. *Hum. Genet.* **4**, 130–5.

194. WALTER, H. and NEMESKÉRI, J. (1969). Populationsgenetische untersuchungen im Brodrogköz (Mo-Ungarn). *Z. Humboldt-Universität zu Berlin, Math.-Nat.* R. XVIII, 885–90.

195. WALTER, H., ARNDT-HANSER, A., RAFFA, M. A., GUMBEL, B. (1975). On the distribution of some genetic markers in Libya. *Hum. Genet.* **27**, 129–36.

196. WELCH, S. G., AIDLEY, D. J., BARRY, J. V., CARTER, N. D., CULLIFORD, B. J., HUNTSMAN, R. B., JENKINS, G. C., POWELL, R. B., and PARR, C. W. (1975). Blood group, serum protein, and red cell enzyme polymorphisms in a population from the Seychelle Islands. *Hum. Hered*. **25**, 346–53.

197. WENDT, G. G., DEICHER, H., and PULS, D. (1963). Die Häufigkeit der Phänotypen des Gammaglobulin-Systems Gm(abxr) und ihre Beziehung zu anderen Erbfaktoren des Blutes. *Z. mensch. Vereb.-u. Konstitutionslehre* **37**, 1–9.

198. WENDT, G. G., ERMERT, A., KIRCHBERG, G., and KINDERMANN, I. (1967). ABO-Blutgruppen und Serumgruppen bei den Negerstämmen Peulh und Marka. *Hum. Genet.* **4**, 74–80.

199. WIEBECKE, D., SPIELMANN, W., and SEIDL, S., (1967). Ein Beitrag zur Populationsgenetik des Gm- and Inv-Systems. *Klin. Wschr.* **45**, 736–7.

200. WIEBECKE, D., DICKHÄUSER, K., and GEOCKE, C. (1969). Die Frequenzen der Gammaglobulin-Serumgruppen Gm(1,2,4,12) und Inv(1) bei Normalpersonen und bei Carcinomträgern. *Bibl. Haemat.* **32**, 64–5.

201. WIEBECKE, D. (1973). Die Frequenzen von Gm(1,2,3,5) und Inv(1) in der Bevölkerung der Bundesrepublik Deutschland. *Hum. Genet.* **18**, 175–80.

MAPS

5 Discussion of the maps

Gm maps

Europe

$Gm^{1,17,21}$

Grubb (1961) noted a cline for Gm(1) in Europe, running from a low value in the south to a higher value in the north. Subsequently (1970) he indicated a west-to-east cline for Gm(-1) (essentially $Gm^{3,5,10,11,13,14,26}$). The isofrequency lines in Map 1, which are based on much more data than those that were available to Grubb, confirm that the south to north cline is supplemented by a west to east cline in southern Europe. The frequency of the $Gm^{1,17,21}$ haplotype is as great in northern Portugal, north-western Spain, and western France as it is in central Scandinavia. There appears also to be a west-east cline in Scandinavia, with $Gm^{1,17,21}$ being most frequent in Norway and north-western Sweden and least frequent in Finland.

$Gm^{1,2,17,21}$

A moderate south-to-north cline for $Gm^{1,2,17,21}$ is apparent (Map 2) but it has broad regions of essentially equal frequencies. There is an interesting 'thrust' of lower frequencies toward the north throughout eastern Europe up to and including Scandinavia. Thus the $Gm^{1,2,17,21}$ haplotype frequencies in eastern and southern Sweden form a trough of lower frequencies between higher frequencies to the east and west.

$Gm^{3,5,10,11,13,14,26}$

The frequency of the $Gm^{3,5,10,11,13,14,26}$ haplotype (Map 3) falls to the north and west from a high plateau value in a region of south-eastern Europe which includes Greece, Albania, Yugoslavia, Bulgaria, Romania, Hungary, and eastern Czechoslovakia (See also Johnson, Kohn, and Steinberg 1977a,b). This distribution is similar to the one for the spread of agriculture from the East into Europe (Menozzi, Piazza, and Cavalli-Svorza 1978; Renfrew 1973). The similarity could lead to the suggestion that the haplotype was introduced from the East, but the $Gm^{3,5,10,11,13,14,26}$ haplotype is uniquely Caucasian, which makes it extremely difficult to accept the East as the haplotype's place of origin.

The populations of eastern and southern Europe have considerable racial admixture, nevertheless the uniquely Caucasoid $Gm^{3,5,10,11,13,14,26}$ haplotype has its highest frequency in precisely this region of Europe. It may be that the haplotype originated in south-eastern Europe; the alternative explanation, that there is strong selection for the haplotype in this region, seems less likely, because no mechanism for such strong selection has been discovered.

Africa (south of the Sahara)

The haplotypes common among Negroids are $Gm^{1,5,10,11,13,14,17,26}$, $Gm^{1,5,10,11,14,17,26}$, $Gm^{1,5,6,11,17,24,26}$, and $Gm^{1,5,6,10,11,14,17,26}$. The first two haplotypes have been combined to form one group (Map 4) and the second two have been combined to form a second group (Map 5). The distribution in southern Africa of $Gm^{1,10,11,13,15,17}$ with or without Gm(16) is shown in Map 6.

Except for the most westerly coastal regions, the $Gm^{1,5,10,11,(13),14,17,26}$ haplotype (Map 4) shows a steady decline in frequency from north to south. Possible explanations are that the haplotype(s) originated in the north or that the pattern is determined by selection. These two explanations are not mutually exclusive and there are no data concerning the appropriateness of either of them.

The $Gm^{1,5,6,(10),11,(14),17,(24),26}$ haplotypes show a plateau of 0.30 at the Anglo–Zambia border region and a decline in frequency to the north and to the south. The distribution strongly suggests that the haplotypes originated in the zone of high frequency, but other explanations are possible. We have noted, as has the reader, that the higher frequencies of the $Gm^{1,5,6,\cdots}$ haplotypes coincide with the region of high frequency of falciparum malaria, of the sickle allele, and of G-6-PD deficiency (reviewed in Allison 1961). This may be, as we suspect, only coincidence.

The $Gm^{1,10,11,13,15,(16),17}$ haplotype is endemic to the Khoisan peoples and has been introduced to Negroids through admixture. It is essentially absent north of Namibia, Botswana, Rhodesia, and Mozambique, but it has been found among Ethiopians (Table XI-4, p. 160). Its frequency increases to the south until it reaches a frequency of 0.25 in the region of Capetown in South Africa. This is probably a reflection of the area of greatest concentration of the Khoisan before the incursion of Caucasoids and Negroids to the region.

The East

Three of the four haplotypes common among Mongoloids ($Gm^{1,17,21}$, $Gm^{1,2,17,21,16}$ and $Gm^{1,10,11,13,15,16,17}$) show a cline of increasing frequency from south to north (Maps 7, 8, and 9). There is also an east to west cline of increasing frequency in the region of Indonesia. Not surprisingly, the $Gm^{1,3,5,10,11,13,14,26}$ haplotype shows clines that are the complement of those for the first three. The $Gm^{1,3,5,10,11,13,14,26}$ haplotype reaches its maximum frequency in the region of Vietnam. Anthropologists and others more familiar with this region of the world than we are may be able to supply information that can help to explain the distribution of these haplotypes.

Papua New Guinea and the Solomon Islands

The $Gm^{1,17,21,26}$ haplotype decreases in a regular cline (Map 11) from a frequency of 0.65 in north-eastern Papua to a freqeuncy of 0.10 to 0.15 in the Solomon Islands to the east. The $Gm^{1,2,17,21,26}$ haplotype on the other hand shows a maximum value in southern New Britain and decreases in frequency to the north and south. The $Gm^{1,2,17,21,26}$ haplotype is essentially absent among those on Papua who speak Melanesian (MN) languages, but it is present among those who speak non-Austronesian (NAN) languages (Giles *et al*. 1965: Schanfield 1971). (See also Tables VI-1, p. 78 and VI-4, p. 84.

The $Gm^{1,5,10,11,13,14,17,26}$ and $Gm^{1,3,5,10,11,13,14,26}$ haplotypes on Papua distinguish the NAN and MN speakers. The former haplotype is more frequent among the NAN speakers than among the MN speakers; the latter haplotype is markedly more frequent among the MN speakers (Steinberg 1967; Schanfield 1971). The clines for these haplotypes are presented in Maps 13 and 14.

The distinctions between MN and NAN speakers with regard to haplotypes are lost on the Solomon Islands, where $Gm^{1,5,10,11,13,14,17,26}$ seems to be completely absent and where $Gm^{1,2,17,21,26}$ is present at low frequency in both language groups (Friedlaender and Steinberg 1970; Steinberg, Damon, and Bloom 1972).

The absence of any distinctions between MN and NAN speakers on the Solomon Islands with respect to haplotype frequencies presents a sharp contrast with the data for such populations on Papua, and raises questions about the origin of the peoples in these two regions. If the MN speakers in both locations had a common origin, we have no explanation for the distinction between those on Papua and those on the Solomon Islands. The same dilemma confronts us concerning the NAN speakers. Almost 50 per cent of them on Papua have the $Gm^{1,5,10,11,13,14,17,26}$ haplotype, but none of them on Bougainville have this haplotype. Possible explanations are founder effect, and selection on the Solomon Islands against the $Gm^{1,5,10,11,13,14,17,26}$ haplotype. It is asking a lot of founder effect to choose a sample, even a relatively small one, lacking $Gm^{1,5,10,11,13,14,17,26}$ from a population in which almost 50 per cent have the haplotype. On the other hand we have no evidence for selection against the haplotype.

Inv maps

The world

Inv[1] plus *Inv*[1,2]

Although only a few populations have been tested for Inv(2), the data indicate that the Inv[1] allele constitutes (with few exceptions) not more than five per cent of the alleles leading to the production of Inv(1). Therefore the data in Map 15 represent essentially the distribution of the *Inv*[1,2] allele. Inv(1) occurs in all populations, hence the map shows the world distribution of the alleles producing it.

The interesting point is that clines are apparent in the Americas, Europe, Africa, and the East. These are, of course, based on fewer data than one would like, but we believe that the clines are real and that larger amounts of data might change details but not the overall picture. It is worth noting that, except for some small regions not indicated in the map, the *Inv*[3] allele occurs with a frequency exceeding 50 per cent in all peoples. We have no explanation to account for the observed distributions.

Bougainville, the Solomon Islands

The clines involve such large areas that they were not apparent during the many investigations involved in gathering the data. A major exception concerns the data for populations on Bougainville (Map 16). Eighteen populations living in villages included within a total distance of about 100 miles were studied for Inv(1) (Friedlaender and Steinberg 1970). They showed a clearly linear cline with the highest frequency of $Gm^{1,(2)}$ (about 0.80) in the north and the lowest frequency (about 0.30) in the south. At a later date, Steinberg *et al*. (1972) studied two more populations on Bougainville (one from the north and one from the south) and three populations on Malaita, about 350 miles to the southeast of Bougainville. The *Inv*[1,(2)] frequencies for the Bougainville samples fit the cline. The frequencies for the Malaita populations fell between 0.20 and 0.25, indicating that the cline may continue across the Solomon Islands. Such a steep cline over so short a range in a region with limited population exchange (Friedlaender 1975) suggests to us that selection of some sort is involved in determining these frequencies, however, see Friedlaender (1975) for another viewpoint.

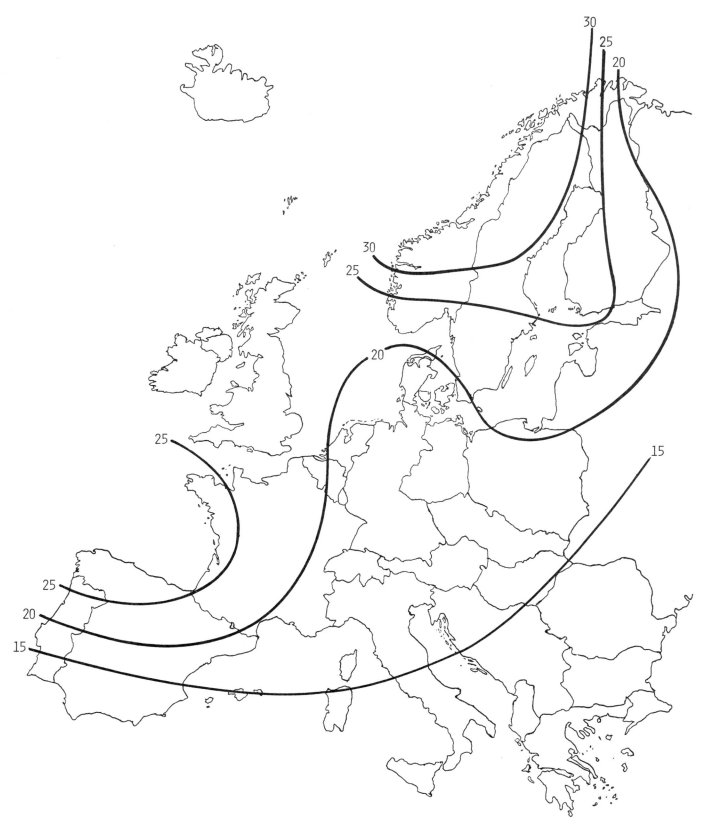

1 Distribution of $Gm^{1,17,21}$ in Europe

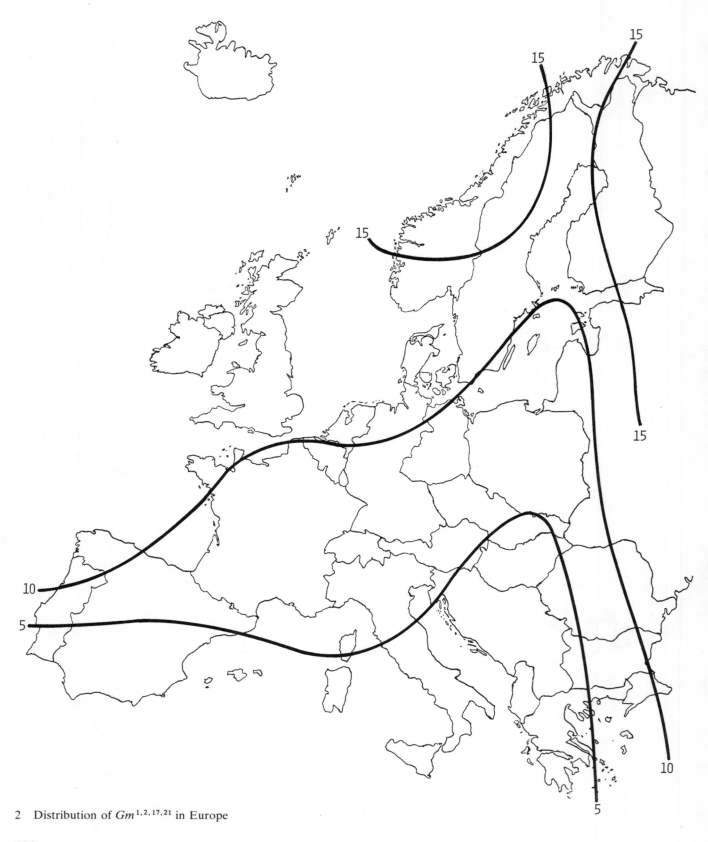

2   Distribution of $Gm^{1,2,17,21}$ in Europe

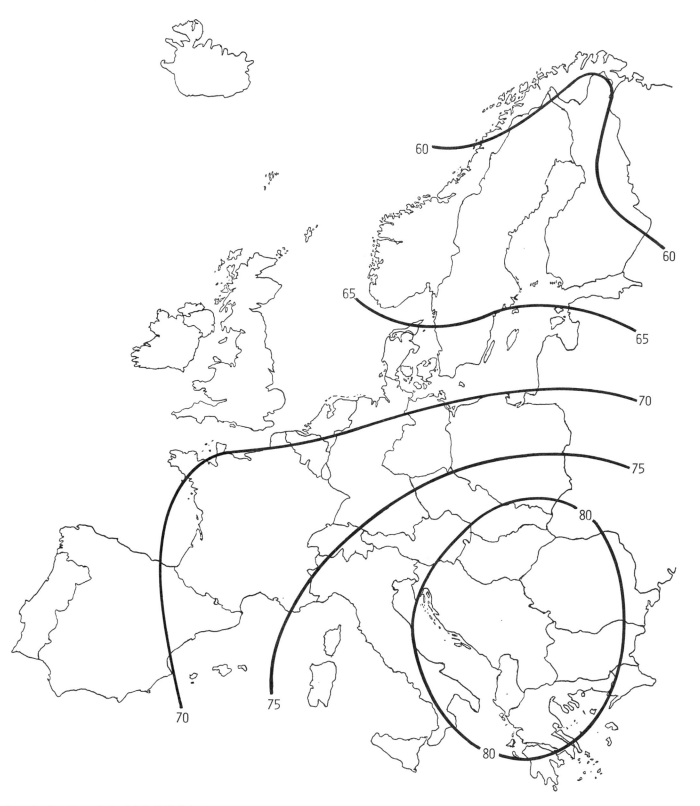

3   Distribution of $Gm^{3,5,10,11,13,14}$ in Europe

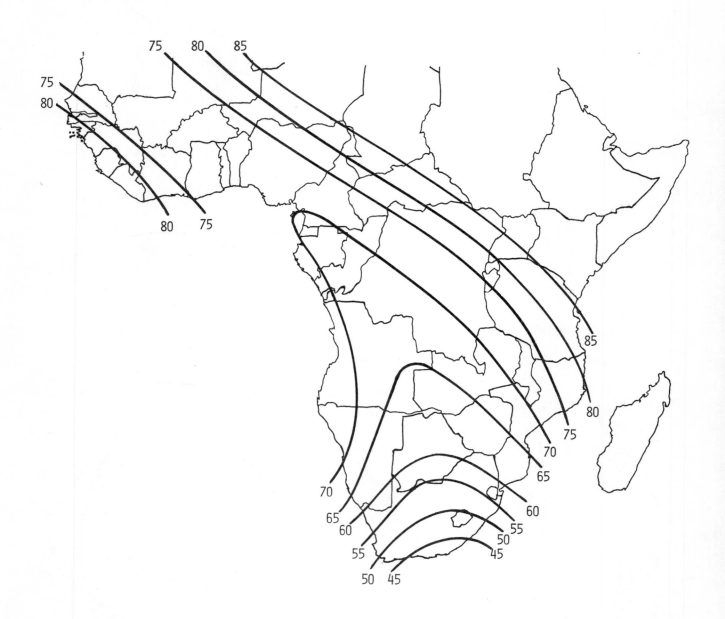

4   Distribution of $Gm^{1,5,10,11,13,14,17}$ in Africa

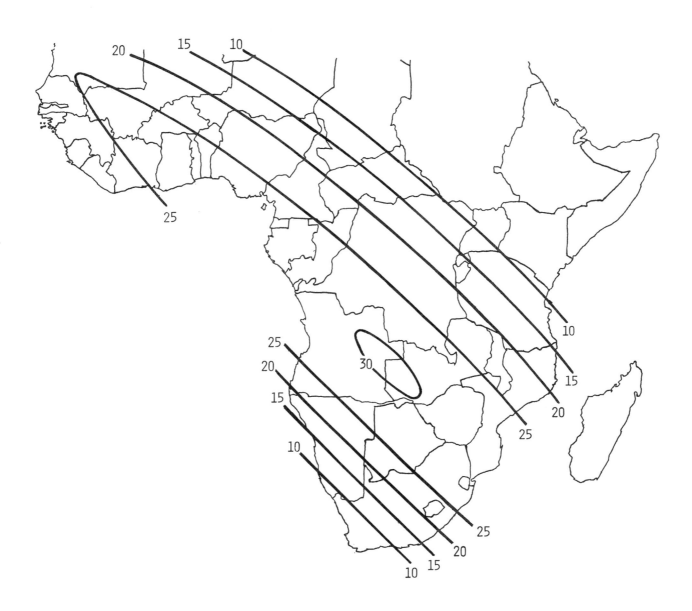

5   Distribution of $Gm^{1,5,6,11,17,24}$ plus $Gm^{1,5,6,10,11,14,17}$ in Africa

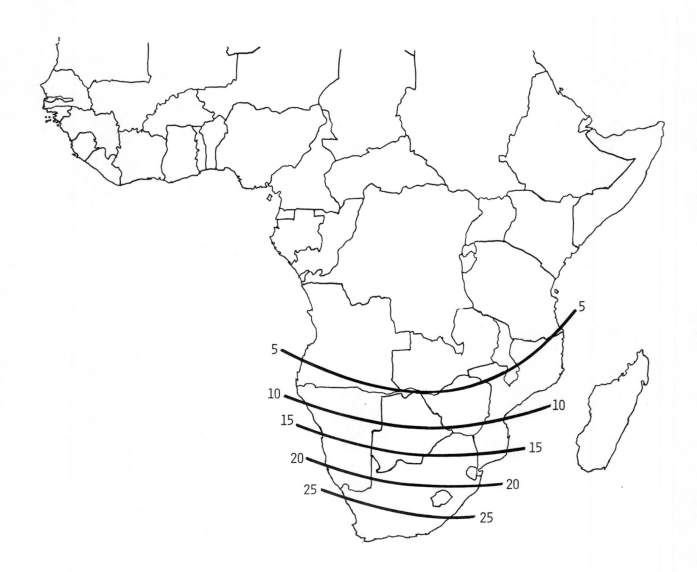

6   Distribution of $Gm^{1,10,11,13,15,17}$ plus $Gm^{1,10,11,13,15,16,17}$ in southern Africa

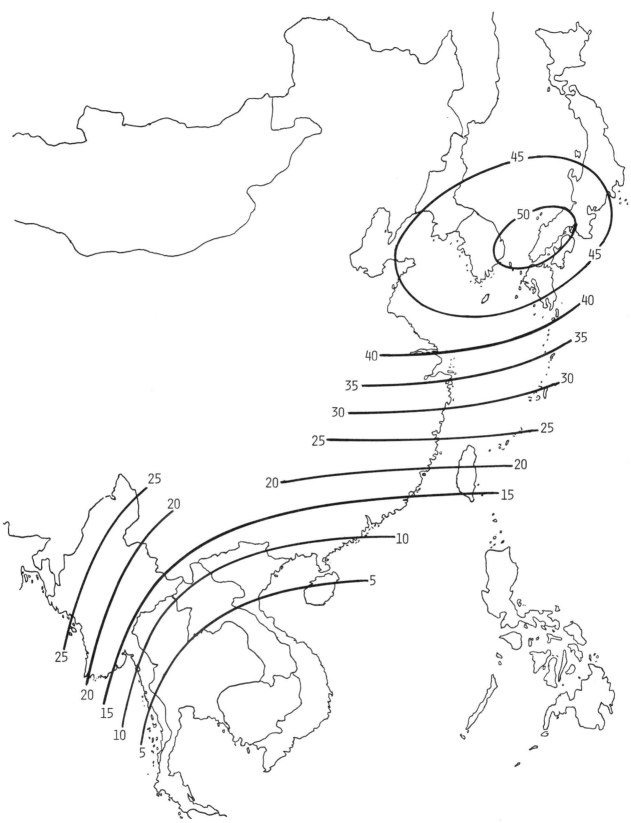

7 Distribution of $GM^{1,17,21}$ in eastern Asia

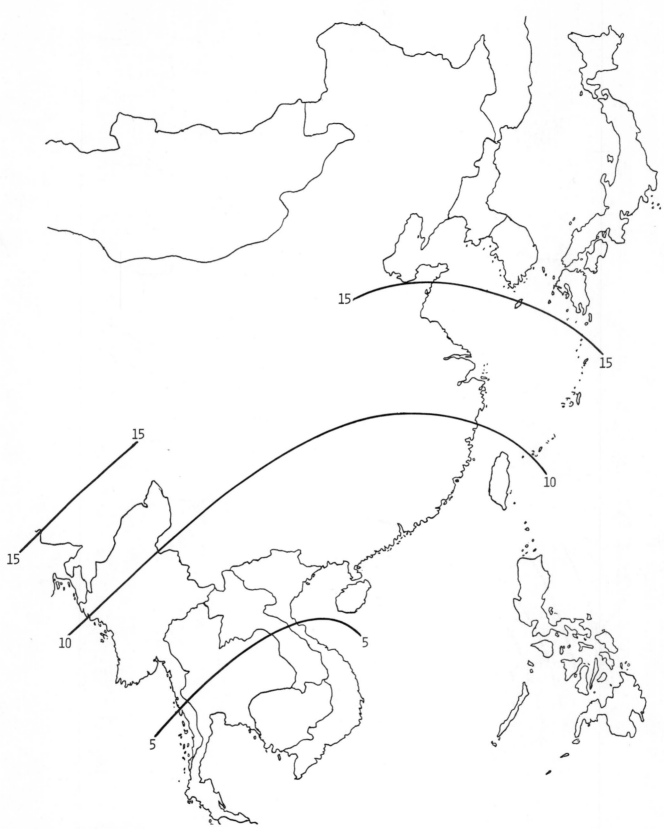

8 Distribution of $Gm^{1,2,17,21}$ in eastern Asia

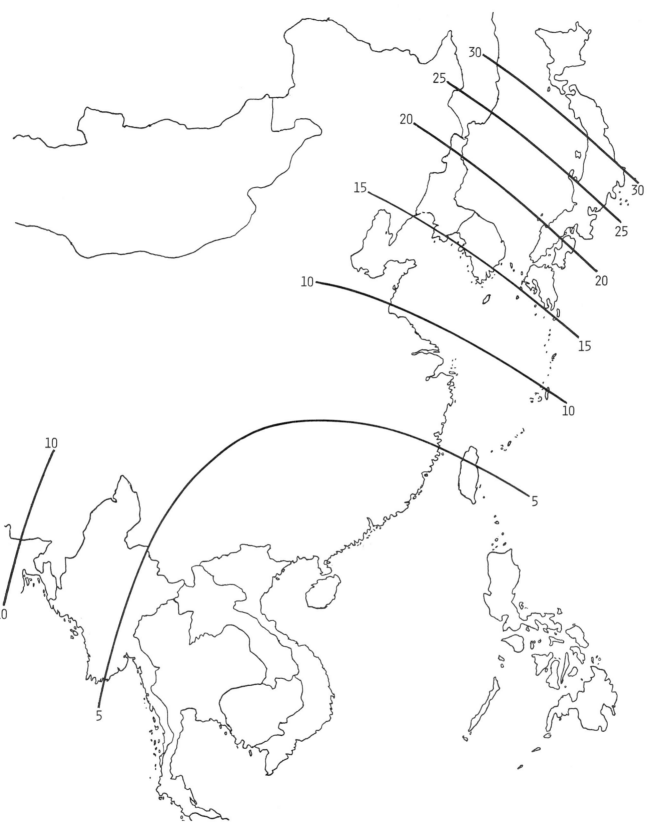

9   Distribution of $Gm^{1, 10, 11, 13, 15, 16, 17}$ in eastern Asia

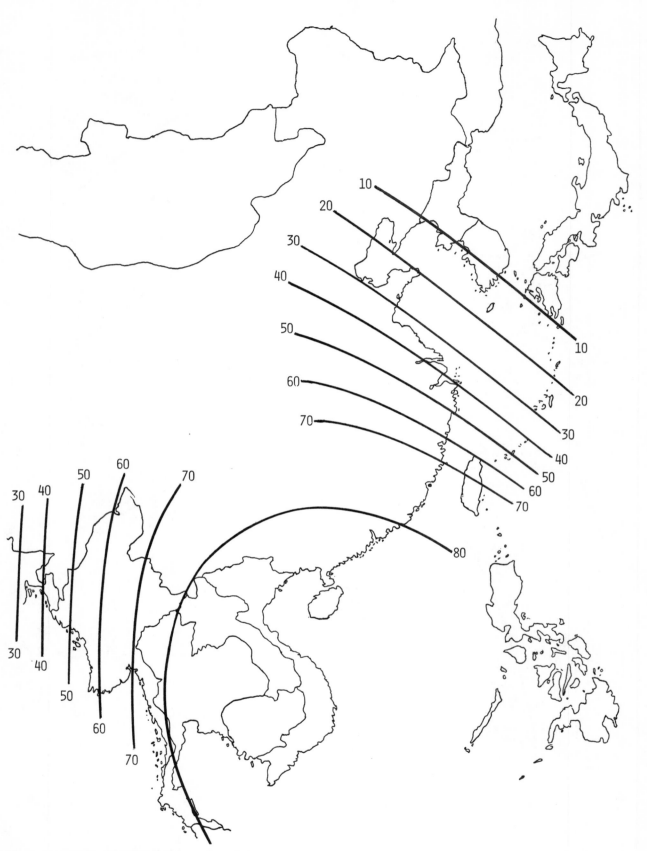

10   Distribution of $Gm^{1,3,5,10,11,13,14}$ in eastern Asia

11 Distribution of *Gm*[1,17,21] in Papua New Guinea and the Solomon Islands

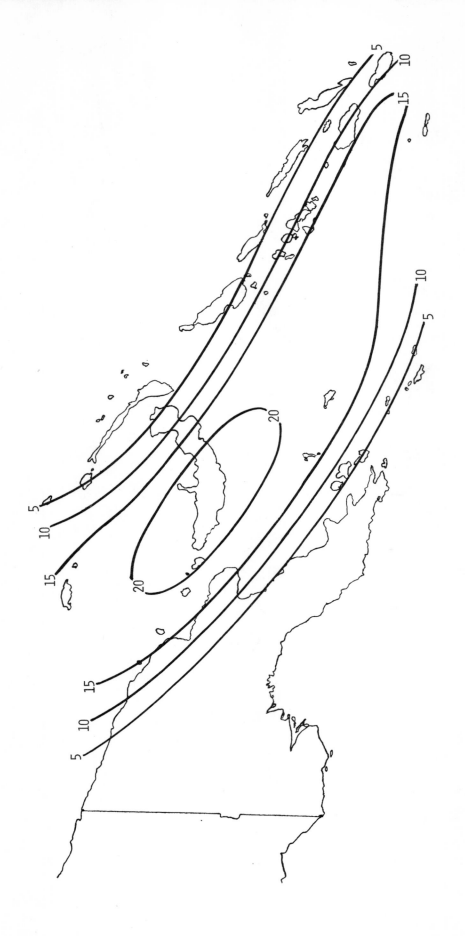

12 Distribution of *Gm*[1,2,17,21] in Papua New Guinea and the Solomon Islands

13   Distribution of $Gm^{1,5,10,11,13,14,17}$ in Papua New Guinea

14 Distribution of $GM^{1,3,5,10,11,13,14}$ in Papua New Guinea and the Solomon Islands

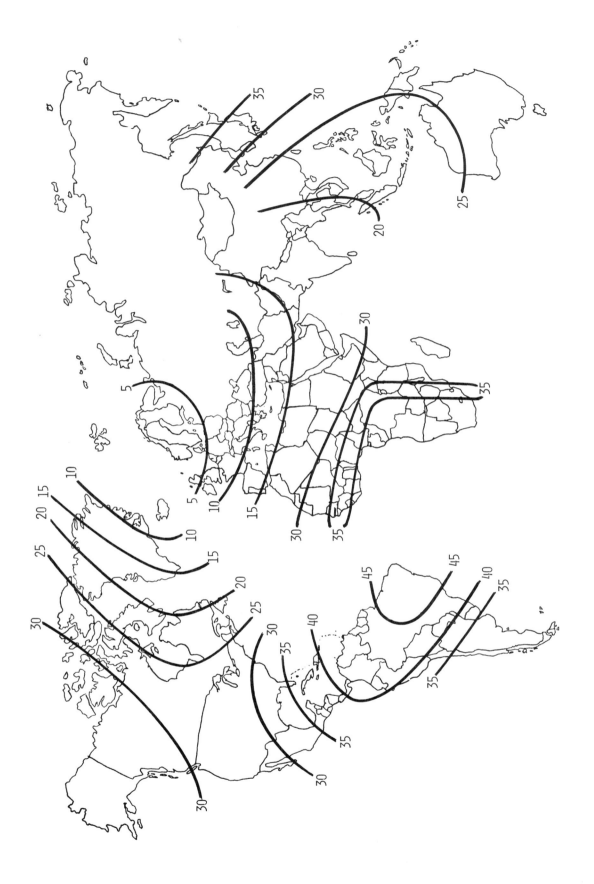

15 Distribution of $INV^{1,2}$ in the world

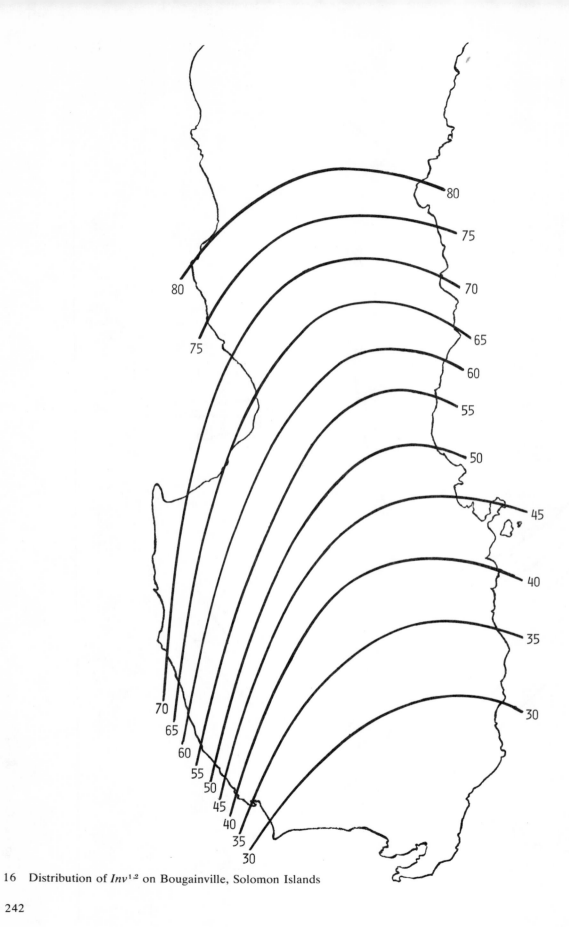

16   Distribution of *Inv*[1,2] on Bougainville, Solomon Islands

Index to tables by continent, country and population

243

OCEANIA – contd.

<small>PAPUA NEW GUINEA</small> – contd.

Bougainville Gm, 80, 81, 82; Inv, 183, 184, 185

Bunamin village Gm, 88; A2m, 214

Eastern Highlands Gm, 79; Inv, 187

Enga NAN Laiagam village Gm, 87; Inv, 188

Fly River Gm, 84; Inv, 186

Gogodara NAN Balimo village Gm, 92; Inv, 188; A2m, 215

Huli, Southern Highlands Gm, 82; Inv, 187

Intoap MN village Gm, 86; Inv, 186

Itsingats MN village Gm, 86; Inv, 185

Karnavitu NAN village Gm, 80; Inv, 183

Kilenge Gm, 84; Inv, 185

Kopani NAN village Gm, 80; Inv, 184

Kopikiri NAN village Gm, 80; Inv, 184

Korpei NAN village Gm, 80; Inv, 184

Koulon village Gm, 88; Inv, 188; A2m, 214

Kuman NAN Minj village Gm, 92; Inv, 188; Inv, 167

Kuraip village Gm, 88; Inv, 188; A2m, 214

Markham Valley Gm, 84; Inv, 186

Moronei NAN village Gm, 81; Inv, 184

Motu MN Porebada village Gm, 93; Inv, 188; A2m, 167

NAN speakers Gm, 78; Inv, 185

Nagovisi NAN Gm, 82; Inv, 185

Nasioi NAN Rumba village Gm, 81; Inv, 185

Nasiwoiwa NAN village Gm, 81; Inv, 184

New Britain Gm, 84, 88, 91; Inv, 185, 188; A2m, 213, 214

New Guinea Gm, 78, 79, 82, 86, 87, 92, 93; Inv, 185, 186, 187, 188; A2m, 215

Nordup village Gm, 91; Inv, 189; A2m, 214

North Fore NAN, eastern highlands Gm, 79; Inv, 187

Nupatoro NAN village Gm, 81; Inv, 184

Okowapaipa NAN village Gm, 81; Inv, 184

Old Siuai NAN village Gm, 81; Inv, 184

Olsobip, Western District Gm, 82; Inv, 187

Onabasula, southern highlands Gm, 82; Inv, 187

Pawaian NAN, eastern highlands Gm, 79

Pomaua NAN village Gm, 81; Inv, 184

Puguap MN village Gm, 86; Inv, 41

Rakunai village Gm, 88; Inv, 188; A2m, 214

Ralmalmal village Gm, 88; A2m, 214

Rorovana MN village Gm, 80; Inv, 183

Rumba NAN village Gm, 81; Inv, 184

Sepik district Gm, 79

Sieronji NAN village Gm, 81; Inv, 184

Simbari NAN, Eastern Highlands Gm, 79

Singas MN village Gm, 86; Inv, 186

South Fore NAN, Eastern Highlands Gm, 79; Inv, 187

Sulka NAN Mope village Gm, 91; A2m, 213

Tench Island Gm, 79

Tolai MN Gm, 88, 91; Inv, 188

Turungum MAN village Gm, 81; Inv, 185

Uruto NAN village Gm, 81; Inv, 185

Usurufa NAN, eastern highlands Gm, 79; Inv, 187

Vairiki village Gm, 88; A2m, 214

Vunalaka village Gm, 88; A2m, 214

Vunalia village Gm, 88; A2m, 214

Waffa NAN, Markham Valley Gm, 84; Inv, 186

Western District Gm, 82; Inv, 187

Yambes, Sepik District Gm, 79

Yanggan NAN, Fly River Gm, 84; Inv, 186

Yanuf MN village Gm, 86; Inv, 186

Yatsing MN village Gm, 86; Inv, 186

<small>SEYCHELLE ISLANDS</small>

Seychelle Islanders Gm, 159; Inv, 209

<small>SOLOMON ISLANDS</small>

Baegu MN Gm, 82; Inv, 189

Bellona Island Gm, 79

Kwaio MN Gm, 82; Inv, 187

Lau MN Gm, 82; Inv, 189

Malaita Gm, 82; Inv, 187, 189

Rennell Island Gm, 79

USA

Filipinos, Honolulu, Hawaii Gm, 103; Inv, 190

Hawaiians, Honolulu, Hawaii Gm, 156; Inv, 208

Honolulu, Hawaii Gm, 103, 156; Inv, 190

SOUTH AMERICA

<small>BOLIVIA</small>

Amantani Indians Gm, 101

Aymara Indians Gm, 98, 101

Chipaya Indians Gm, 98; Inv, 190

Guaqui Indians Gm, 101

Lake Titicaca Gm, 101

Llachon Indians Gm, 101

Mocetenes Indians Gm, 98

Pecheurs Indians Gm, 98

Puno Indians Gm, 101

Quechua Indians Gm, 98

Taquile Indians Gm, 101

<small>BRAZIL</small>

Aweikoma Indians, Santa Catarina Gm, 103; Inv, 196

Caingang Indians, Santa Catarina Gm, 103; Inv, 197

Caingang Mestizos, Santa Catarina Gm, 103; Inv, 197

Cayapo Indians Gm, 118; Inv, 196

Guarini Indians, Santa Catarina Gm, 103; Inv, 197

Kuben-Kran-Kegn Gm, 118; Inv, 196

Mato Grosso Gm, 104

Mekranoti Gm, 118; Inv, 196

Santa Catarina Gm, 103; Inv, 196, 197

Sao Domingos Gm, 112

Sao Marcos Gm, 112; Inv, 197

Simoes Lopes Gm, 112; Inv, 197

Txukahamae Gm, 118; Inv, 196

Xavante Indians Gm, 112

Xavante Indians, Mato Grosso Gm, 104

Xavante Indians, Sao Marcos Inv, 197

Xavante Indians, Simoes Lopes Inv, 197

Xikrin Gm, 118; Inv, 196

<small>FRENCH GUIANA</small>

Emerillon Indians Gm, 99, 131; Inv, 201

Galibi Indians Gm, 99

Maroni Gm, 131; Inv, 201

Oayana Indians Gm, 99

Oyampi Indians Gm, 99

Oyampi Indians, Oyapok Gm, 131; Inv, 201

Oyapok Gm, 131; Inv, 201

Palikoar Indians Gm, 99

Wayana Indians, Maroni Gm, 131; Inv, 201

<small>PARAGUAY</small>

Ayore Indians Gm, 104; Inv, 197

Cheroti Indians Gm, 104; Inv, 197

Chulupi Indians Gm, 104; Inv, 197

Guarayu Indians Gm, 104; Inv, 197

Guayaki Indians Gm, 104; Inv, 198

Lengua Indians Gm, 104; Inv, 197

North-West Gm, 104; Inv, 197, 198

Sanapana Indians Gm, 104; Inv, 198

South West Gm, 104; Inv, 198

Tapiete Indians Gm, 104; Inv, 198

Toba Indians Gm, 104; Inv, 198

<small>SURINAM</small>

Bush Negro A2m, 217

Non-Paramaribo regions Gm, 144

Paramaribo regions Gm, 144

Trio Indians Gm, 132; Inv, 198

Wajana Indians Gm, 132; Inv, 198

<small>VENEZUELA</small>

Paraujano Indians Gm, 99; Inv, 198

Piaroa Indians Inv, 198

Waica Indians Inv, 198

Index to tables by population